the
Smoke Free
diet

the Smoke Free diet

Waist Away and Kick Those Butts!

Bradley Burnam

Table of Contents

Introduction   vii

Chapter One: The Costs of Addiction   1

Chapter Two: The Chemistry of Addiction   7

Chapter Three: The Psychology of Addiction   11

Chapter Four: How and Why the Smoke Free Diet
Works   15

Chapter Five: Time to Waist Away and Kick Those
Butts   27

Chapter Six: Dietary Supplements   37

Chapter Seven: A Lifelong Eating Plan for the
Addictive Personality   49

Chapter Eight: Exercise: Fit from the Inside-Out   53

Chapter Nine: Final Tips to Beef Up Your Arsenal   63

Appendix A: Easy and Savory Low-carb Recipes   67

Appendix B: Mini Carb Counter   81

Introduction

What if I told you that you no longer need fear the likely reality of weight gain while quitting smoking? What if I went a step further and told you that you could lose weight, increase muscle tone, increase energy, and lower your cholesterol, blood pressure, and triglyceride levels, all *while* you were quitting? What if I told you that the dietary regimen this book prescribes is already one of the most widely employed weight-loss and maintenance programs in history? What if I also told you that the psychological and biochemical mechanisms activated by this diet quite literally mimic the previously nearly unbreakable addictions that smoking creates? Would you believe me? You will.

To be honest, it is quite surprising to me that these dietary principles, which have been in existence and widely employed for decades, have never been applied to smoking cessation. After reading this book, the physiological and psychological synergies will seem obvious. As I said, the proof that this diet will strip pounds of fat off you already exists. In fact, the eating regimen that will help you quit smoking while simultaneously losing weight and rapidly stabilizing all of your vitals (blood pressure, cholesterol, and triglycerides) occupies at least a shelf in nearly every bookstore in this country. Moreover, there are now pre-made, nutritionally appropriate foods of every type, size, color, and texture, as well as web sites, licensed experts, and support groups...it is a multi-billion dollar industry even while I write this book. While I will explain how the prescribed dietary regimen works in plain Engilsh, my sales pitch for its effectiveness as a weight loss tool has long-since been completed. *What I will sell you on, however, is the physical and psychological synergy between these eating principles and smoking cessation that you can take advantage of right now*; but, for that, you must read on.

Now, I won't insult your intelligence by telling you that smoking is bad for you; I will make the logical jump that reading this book is proof enough that you are, at least, contemplating quitting and fundamentally know why you should. But quitting is hard. Nicotine is addictive, among the most addictive substances on the planet. Moreover, *the physical act of smoking engenders psychological addictions that must be broken, including the fear of weight gain.* When you tried to quit last time and just couldn't resist stopping by the gas station to pick up one more pack, it was not weakness; it was chemistry joining forces with psychology, and they are a tough duo to battle with...but they are not invincible. **The beauty of this diet is that it addresses both of these quitting road blocks: the biochemical addiction created by nicotine use *and* the psychological addictions, including the fear of weight gain, created by the physical act of smoking.**

In this book, you will learn with absolute certainty that weight gain need not be an inevitable consequence of quitting. You will learn *why* you are addicted to smoking, as well as how eating in the manner prescribed mimics and replaces both the chemical and psychological addictions, thus enabling you to break free of both bonds. You will learn how the diet works in terms of weight loss and the rapid stabilization of your vitals, (cholesterol, blood pressure, and triglycerides), as well as how to incorporate the eating plan into your daily life. You will learn lifelong dietary and fitness techniques designed to prevent relapse. Finally, you will be smoke free, and that is the greatest finale of all.

Chapter One

The Costs of Addiction

So, I promised not to insult your intelligence by telling you that smoking is bad for you, but I never promised I wouldn't tell you just how bad it is for you, both physiologically and economically. No self-respecting book on smoking cessation should be without at least a brief chapter on the health and economic costs of smoking addiction.

You're Not Alone

Believe it or not, the majority of American adults have had some experience with nicotine. According to a survey conducted all the way back in 1997 by the National Institute on Drug Abuse, approximately 71 percent of the population, age twelve or older, had tried at least a few puffs of a cigarette at some point in their lives; according to this same report, approximately 33 percent of the population had smoked a cigarette during the past year. The 1999 National Household Survey on Drug Abuse showed that an estimated fifty-seven million Americans were current smokers, a statistic that placed nicotine squarely among the most abused substances on Earth. In addition, this same survey reported that, in 1998, each day in the United States, more than two thousand people under the age of eighteen began daily smoking; by 2010, the Center for Disease Control estimated that 25 percent of US high school students were regular smokers. As of today, over 20 percent of the US and global population smoke regularly. So, again, you're not alone.

The impact of nicotine addiction in terms of morbidity and mortality is staggering. Tobacco kills more than 430,000 US citizens each year, more than alcohol, cocaine, heroin, homicide, suicide, car accidents, fire, and AIDS combined. Tobacco use is the leading preventable cause of death in the United States and takes credit for one of every five total deaths; if you're quitting for a loved one, know that secondhand inhalation is consistently ranked near the top, as well, so he/she will be grateful.

4000 Chemicals in One Little Stick?

That's right...tobacco smoke contains over four thousand chemicals, at least sixty-three of which have been linked to cancer in humans (not just lab rats...humans). It's not just your lungs, either; there's cancer of the lungs, lips, tongue, throat, esophagus, pharynx, stomach, pancreas, bladder, cervix, ureter, and kidneys, as if one weren't enough. Basically, just about every major organ of your body gets hit by each puff, either directly or indirectly, and these "hits" lead to damage and, thus, cancerous cell growth.

A Detailed Look at Some of the Worst Offenders

Nicotine: You will learn all you ever wanted to know about nicotine, one of the most addictive substances on Earth, in the next chapter, but did you know that nicotine is also used as a common insecticide?

Carbon Monoxide (CO): It comes out of your car's tail-pipe (unless you managed to get your hands on a hydro-gen-powered car before the rest of us). When you inhale carbon monoxide, your red blood cells, which are designed to transport oxygen to your organs, actually choose the carbon monoxide instead. Red blood cells are your body's boxcars for oxygen; carbon monoxide locks the doors to these cars. Result: Less oxygen to your organs and in-creased risk of heart attack and/or stroke.

Tar: Nearly identical to the black stuff on which you drove to work. However, unlike on the freeway, there are tiny little structures in your lungs called cilia, which act as the cleaning service for your respiratory system twen-ty-four hours per day. Tar from cigarettes sticks to your cilia, making them unable to carry out their assignments. Airways fill with mucus, leading to that ever-so-attractive smoker's cough. You become far more susceptible to air-borne contaminants, even germs. Eventually, your lungs become scarred from their inability to filter contaminants and unable to get enough oxygen into the bloodstream (keep in mind that the red blood cells are already lacking oxygen due to the carbon monoxide). Have you ever seen somebody toting around an oxygen tank with wheels? Chances are very high that he/she was/is a smoker.

Hydrogen Cyanide: This chemical serves multiple purposes in modern and premodern society. It's in your cigarettes, as well as gas chambers. Enough said.

Statistically speaking, tobacco use accounts for one-third of all cancers, period. Foremost among the cancers caused by tobacco is lung cancer, the number one cancer killer of both men and women. Cigarette smoking has been linked to approximately 90 percent of all lung cancer cases.

In addition to lung cancer, smoking causes lung diseases such as chronic bronchitis and emphysema, and has been found to exacerbate asthma symptoms in adults and children, whether by primary or secondary ingestion. The overall rates of death from cancer are twice as high among smokers as nonsmokers, with heavy smokers having rates that are four times greater than those of nonsmokers. Cigarette smoking is the most prevalent, preventable cause of cancer in the United States.

Cigarette smoking was first reported to have a relationship with coronary heart disease in the 1940s. Since that time, it has been well documented that smoking substantially increases the risk of heart disease, including stroke, heart attack, vascular disease, and aneurysms. It is estimated that nearly one-fifth of deaths from heart disease are attributable to smoking.

We tend to focus primarily on health effects stemming from the direct use of cigarettes, but as briefly mentioned above, those of you who smoke around loved ones should know that secondhand smoke increases the risk for many diseases. Environmental tobacco smoke (ETS) is a major source of indoor air contaminants; secondhand smoke is estimated to cause approximately three thousand lung cancer deaths per year among nonsmokers and contributes to as many as forty thousand deaths related to cardiovascular disease. Exposure to tobacco smoke in the home increases the severity of asthma for children and is a risk factor for new cases of childhood asthma. ETS exposure has also been linked with "sudden infant death syndrome."

The *Cost* of Smoking

I'm no mathematician, so I'll keep this brief and straightforward. How much money would you save if you quit today?

If each pack averages, say, six dollars, and you smoke one pack per day, that's 42 dollars per week, 168 dollars per month, and 2016 dollars per year. Over twenty years, barring inflation, that's a hell of a nice car, or condo, or private hut on a beach in Bora Bora! Now, to you heavy smokers out there, multiply that by three or four and you've got your kids' college tuition (or, a really, really nice car, or boat, or multistory hut in Bora Bora with private butler). Give yourself a little extra motivation and start planning the way you'll spend that extra cash once you've completed the Smoke Free Diet.

A Light at the End of the Chapter

There is good news: following the Smoke Free Diet and ridding yourself of your habit will drastically improve not just your finances but your health, no matter how long you've been smoking. Research has shown that, for the average smoker, within two weeks of quitting, coughing, congestion, lethargy, and shortness of breath decrease; overall energy increases, and walking no longer becomes a task. Between the one-month and nine-month mark, the lung cilia regenerate, and consequently the shortness of breath further decreases. Within one year, your risk of heart disease will be half that of a smoker. Within five years, you will decrease your chance of lung cancer by half, and within ten to fifteen years, your precancerous cells will have been replaced and your risk of dying from cancer will be similar to that of someone who has never smoked.

Chapter Two
The Chemistry of Addiction

What Is Nicotine?

Nicotine, while one of more than four thousand chemicals found in cigarette smoke, is the primary component in tobacco that acts on the brain. It is also, as stated above, recognized as one of the most frequently used and addictive drugs on the planet. But what does nicotine look like? It is a naturally occurring, colorless liquid that turns brown when burned and acquires the odor of tobacco when exposed to air. Since nicotine was first identified in the early eighteen hundreds, it has been studied extensively and shown to have a number of complex and sometimes unpredictable effects on the brain and the body.

Most cigarettes in the U.S. market contain at least ten milligrams (mg) of nicotine, and through inhalation the average smoker takes in one to two mg of nicotine per cigarette. Nicotine is absorbed not just through the lungs, but through the skin and mucosal lining of the mouth and nose. Cigarettes are, in fact, nothing more than a highly engineered, highly effective drug delivery system; nicotine reaches the brain within just ten seconds of inhalation! Now, the average smoker will take ten puffs from a cigarette over a period of five minutes. Do the math: a person who smokes one pack (twenty cigarettes) daily gets two hundred highly addictive slaps in the cranium per day.

Is Nicotine Addictive?

If the Marlboro Man could speak clearly through his oxygen mask, he'd likely agree: nicotine *is* highly addictive. Addiction is characterized by compulsive drug seeking and use, even in the face of negative health consequences, and tobacco use more than fits this bill. It is well documented that the majority of smokers identify tobacco as harmful and express a desire to reduce or stop using it, and nearly thirty-five million of them make a serious attempt to quit each year. *Unfortunately, less than 7 percent of those who try to quit on their own achieve more than one year of abstinence; most relapse within a few days of attempting to quit.* Are you ready to break that trend?

Recent research has shown in even finer detail exactly how nicotine acts on the brain. Of primary importance to its addictive nature, as well as to our task in this book, are findings that nicotine activates the brain circuitry that regulates feelings of pleasure, or, the so-called "reward pathways." A key brain chemical involved in regulating and provoking the desire to consume drugs is the neurotransmitter **dopamine**; research has shown that nicotine drastically increases the levels of dopamine in the reward circuitry of the brain *(Keep this in mind, as this* "dopaminergic" circuitry is a foundational principal of the Smoke Free Diet). Interestingly, nicotine can simultaneously stimulate and relax you-that's why people find reason to smoke in times of anger or glee. But the acute effects of nicotine (increased blood pressure, respiration, and heart rate, along with the associated adrenaline surge) dissipate in a few minutes, causing the smoker to continue dosing frequently throughout the day to maintain the drug's pleasurable effects and prevent withdrawal.

How Does Nicotine Deliver Its Effect?

Immediately after exposure to nicotine, nicotine causes a release of dopamine in the brain regions that control pleasure and motivation, or the reward pathways. There is an associated "kick" and rush of adrenaline, which stimulates the body and causes a sudden increase in blood pressure, respiration, and heart rate. This reaction is similar to that caused by other drugs, such as cocaine, heroin, and amphetamines, and is thought to underlie the pleasurable sensations experienced by many smokers. Important to note for later, in addition to increasing brain dopamine levels, nicotine suppresses insulin output from the pancreas. Insulin is, safe to say, one of the most (if not the most) influential hormones in the body for weight, mood, and energy balance...and we will delve into it in great detail. But know this in advance: your habit may have prepared you for the reduction in insulin that the Smoke Free Diet brings about; in essence, you will more than likely have an easier adjustment to the prescribed eating plan than a nonsmoker.

What Happens after Long-term Use of Nicotine?

Chronic exposure to nicotine results in addiction, plain and simple. Repeated exposure to nicotine results in the development of a tolerance, or a state in which higher doses of a drug are required to produce the same stimulating effects as earlier doses. Long-term nicotine use produces such a tolerance and the physiologic effects can be quite profound. But, keep in mind that, on a short-term basis, nicotine is metabolized fairly rapidly, disappearing from the body only a few hours after that last puff; therefore, an acute tolerance (one created between morning and night) will also be created, and some of it is lost overnight, which is why smokers often report that their first cigarettes of the day are the strongest and/or the "best." The flip side of this is that, since nicotine is metabolized quickly, your body can begin to repair the acute damage quickly. As stated in the last chapter, your body is a very efficient repair shop.

Chapter Three

The Psychology of Addiction

When I wrote the first draft of *The Smoke Free Diet,* I lumped the chemistry and psychology of addiction into one chapter entitled "Why You're Addicted." Upon further thought, I realized that the psychology of smoking addiction deserves a volume of books, let alone its own chapter.

Truthfully, how many of you woke up one morning and said, "My dopaminergic feedback system just isn't doing the trick anymore...I should start smoking"? Unless you're a practicing neuroscientist with very powerful measures of self-awareness (all the way down to the synapses), I would venture to say that something else led you to your habit. Was it peer pressure, advertising, modeling your parents' behavior...maybe that action hero puffing away while saving the world? Whatever it was, it was psychological. One or all of these motivational factors affected your psyche, and you took your first puff, then your second, and so on.

Today, when you pick up a cigarette, will it be a conscious attempt to increase the dopamine level in your brain, to appease the reward circuitry? No? So, why do you smoke? I'm certain that your current list of reasons does not match the initial reasons behind your lighting up, whenever that was; you are probably older, wiser, and less concerned with the image that smoking gives you, an image that is gradually becoming less attractive, I might add. Let's make a list of reasons, at least one or more of which should fit every reader, as to why you continue to smoke:

Emotional
1. Stress reduction
2. Relaxation
3. Decreases boredom and/or loneliness
4. Feeling depressed when you don't (byproduct of dopamine reduction in the brain)
5. Alleviates anxiety

Situational
1. Comfortable distraction in social situations
2. Task-based; increases focus/concentration
3. Your friends are
4. After a meal
5. Morning ritual
6. Coffee or tea consumption
7. Alcohol consumption
8. Last thing you do before going to bed
9. Stops you from eating

Let's give this list of reasons a name, "triggers," and face some facts: you're not just addicted to the chemicals in that cigarette; you're addicted to the triggers, as well. **Being without a cigarette in any of these situations, emotional or social, can make withdrawal symptoms or cravings worse.** While nicotine gum and patches, and even the newer and somewhat effective (and unbelievably expensive) pill-form agents, may pharmacologically alleviate the biochemical aspects of withdrawal, cravings often persist that stem from the psychological underpinnings of your addiction. In these areas, such quitting agents offer no aid, but the Smoke Free Diet actually replaces and eliminates them.

It's very important that you examine your own list of triggers, no matter how lengthy it may be; recognition of the situations that lead to cravings is important, as you may wish to avoid as many of them as possible while kicking the habit (obviously, you can't avoid sleeping, but you can make less trips to the coffeehouse or bar down the street before hitting the sack). In truth, it is highly unlikely that any of the above triggers happened for the first time while you had a cigarette in your mouth; you created the association, and because of this, you have the power to eliminate it. But, for those situations you can't avoid, emotional or social (and, even the ones you can, but choose not to), fear not...the Smoke Free Diet addresses, replaces, and eliminates these situationally dependent cravings, not just biochemically, but psychologically. For those of you who smoke to eliminate food cravings or to lose weight, after reading the next chapter, you'll realize that you're in for the greatest "treat" of them all, because you're about to find out that you can eat as much as you want, as often as you want, and drop weight by the kilo.

Chapter Four

How and Why the Smoke Free Diet Works

In order to understand how the Smoke Free Diet will enable you to quit smoking once and for all, it is first necessary to understand how it will, simultaneously, drop unwanted pounds and stabilize your vitals (cholesterol, blood pressure, and triglycerides).

The principle behind the Smoke Free Diet is a controlled carbohydrate approach to eating. Other authors have spent hundreds of pages *attempting* to describe the scientific principles behind weight loss and the low-carbohydrate lifestyle (and I've read every single page and more); I'll sum up the science for you in a few paragraphs, which, at the risk of sounding insulting to my colleagues, is all that is necessary to understand it.

For those of you who always wanted to be scientists, you're in luck; I want you to conduct a very simple experiment using three ingredients that you almost certainly have in your kitchen, along with a clear drinking glass. If you don't feel like getting out of bed, just take my word for it.

Pour a glass of water about half full. Next, pour some oil (cooking oil is fine) on the top. What happened? Like the cliché says, oil and water didn't mix. Now, pour some sugar in the glass with the oil and water. What happened? Gradually, the oil falls and mixes into the water. You've just proved that the controlled-carbohydrate approach to eating works.

The water in this experiment represents the plasma content of your blood which, coincidentally, is mostly water. The oil (fats) and sugar (carbohydrates) are being introduced one at a time by you, just as if you were eating them. But, just like in the glass, no matter how much you eat, fat cannot enter the bloodstream without carbohydrates, plain and simple. No carbohydrates...no fat absorption. Byproduct: eating in a controlled-carbohydrate manner turns your body into a fat-burning furnace twenty-four hours per day, as stored bodyfat is the second most usable source of energy behind carbohydrates. More on that in a moment...

There is one other chemical that can't be illustrated in this experiment but plays an important role in the fat-burning and smoking-cessation equation: insulin. Insulin is a hormone secreted by the pancreas in response to rises in blood sugar; its primary intention in the hopeful homeostasis that is your body is to lower blood sugar back to normal, resting levels. But insulin has multiple personalities and multiple effects; in its other life, it is a metaphorical "taxi" for fat storage, or a "router" hormone.

However, insulin release is at your mercy; your pancreas will not secrete insulin unless you consume carbohydrates. So without carbohydrates, any fat that you consume can whistle for that taxi hormone all day and night, but it will not get a ride to the storage yard, otherwise known as your stomach, thighs, or rear end.

Another factor that comes into play is something called bioavailability. What this means, in everyday terms, is how chemically available something is to your body for usage. Carbohydrate consumption elevates blood sugar, and blood sugar is the most biologically available source of energy for your body. What is the second most bio-logically available source (hint...go back a couple para-graphs)? You guessed it: stored bodyfat. Your body only has two days' worth of sugar stored up in its liver as a substance called glycogen; after two days without carbo-hydrates, this supply gets depleted and your body must, instead, turn to stored fat for energy. This biochemical changeover takes about forty-eight hours and the state you achieve in which your body utilizes fat for energy is called ketosis. When you enter this state of ketosis, you will burn stored fat at an astonishing rate twenty-four hours per day, which is described in the next paragraph.

A concept not done sufficient literary justice by other books on the controlled-carbohydrate approach to eat-ing is the basal metabolic rate, or, BMR. The BMR is how many calories your body burns every day just existing; that's right...your body is burning calories as you read. Your heart burns calories beating; your fingers burn calo-ries on that remote control. Even just sitting all day burns, on average, over a thousand calories, and far more than that if you weigh more than you should...even more than that if you have notable muscle tone, as muscle burns calories to sustain its existence. Overweight people burn thousands of calories per day just breathing and sitting. But if you have no blood sugar available for your body to burn, *it must burn fat to exist.* I know this may sound too good to be true, but *eating no carbohydrates means that you will burn fat just by existing.* When you consider that each pound of fat has roughly 3200 calories of stored energy in it, you can burn pounds per week just by altering your eating habits. If you exercise to top it off, you can lose weight at a rate that will astonish you.

What this all boils down to in the weight-loss and, consequently, vitals-reduction paradigm is the following simple equation: you can consume as much food as you want, as long as you reduce your carbohydrate intake significantly. The Smoke Free Diet will enable you to eat unrestricted quantities of satisfying and delicious foods as often as you want, as long as you eat correctly...and it always works; your body was designed that way. *The only way that the controlled-carbohydrate approach can fail is if you cheat or unknowingly eat carbohydrates.* Examples of unexpected carb sources include condiments (ketchup and barbeque sauce), salad dressings (check the label), even an innocent breast of chicken coated in sugary terriyaki sauce can yank you right out of that blissful and productive state that is twenty-four-hour-per-day fat burning, or, ketosis. Have no fear...you will be armed with the tools to prevent such errors via the acceptable food lists provided. But let's take some time to examine carbohy-drates at a biochemical level, giving you the opportunity to learn a great deal more about what you will be avoid-ing; once you know all the facts, you will feel less like you are shunning an old friend and more as if you are kicking out that leech of a roommate who stopped paying rent years ago, but keeps taking up more and more space.

So, what the *devil* is a carbohydrate? To your weight and mood, with the exception of select "good carbs," which I'll talk about in a moment, the italicized word in the last sentence is quite fitting. Chemically speaking, however, what is a carbohydrate?

While there are different types of carbohydrates, to the body there is little difference between any carbohy-drate-containing foods at the biochemical level. Bread and candy have extremely similar effects on body chemistry, the primary difference being the time they take to digest and the speed at which you release insulin. Carbohydrates are chains of molecules. "Complex" carbohydrates, like those contained in bread, pasta, potatoes, and starches are the lengthier chains and take longer for your diges-tive system to process than simple carbohydrates (candy, table sugar, etc.). This legthier digestion time results in a slower release of insulin and less of the fleeting "spike" in mood, energy, and anxiety caused by a rapid release of insulin. Moreover, with less of a spike comes less of a crash, with the accompanying fatigue, irritability, and rapid onset of hunger to follow. Science lesson aside, for our purposes, a carbohydrate is a sugar and a sugar is a carbohydrate.

There are, as I have said, some "good carb" foods with extremely low carb counts that are allowed during the program (such as green vegetables); as you reach your target weight and begin the lifelong eating plan, the quantities will be increased and more variety will be introduced. However, "good carbs" is a more complicated concept than it sounds. For something to be a good carbohydrate, it must first of all have a very low glycemic index, or speed of digestion (way, way lower than candy-coated, simple carbs). Second, it must have a low caloric density, which means that, pound for pound, it must have very few calories compared to other carbohydrate-containing foods. Comparing strawberries (forty calories and ten carbs per cup) and pasta (four hundred calories and over forty grams of carbs per cup) illustrates this point very well. Typically, foods that fit into the good carb category are also high in fiber (i.e., broccoli).

Fiber is an interesting compound because it is defined as a carbohydrate but has no effect on blood sugar; *you can subtract fiber from total carbohydrates on any nutrition label to determine the "net carb count."* A few more examples of good carbs are spinach (very high in fiber with a low caloric density), mushrooms (extremely low caloric density), and nearly the entire berry family (very high in fiber and low caloric density). *However, in the initial phase of this diet, the one that you follow until you succeed in quitting, it is highly recommended that you limit your intake of even good carbs to ten or less grams per day (not including fiber), and if possible spread this over multiple meals.* To make this less daunting, detailed carb counts and serving sizes will be provided later in the book. When you have both quit and reached your target weight and therefore are ready to progress to the lifelong eating plan outlined in chapter six, you can gradually add more of these foods back to your daily ritual; you won't be giving up all carbohydrates forever. As I will explain in the next chapter, during the quitting phase, I want you to *shoot* for little to no carbohydrates while in reality never exceeding twenty grams per day. It is nearly impossible to consume zero carbohydrates, as even some meats contain trace amounts of carbohydrates, but it's better to shoot for zero and expect sub-twenty than to shoot for twenty and end up over the limit.

So, how does the controlled-carbohydrate approach to eating, in addition to stripping fat and stabilizing your vitals, alleviate the chemical and psychological withdrawals of smoking cessation? It comes down to one, simple, all-encompassing, beautiful concept: *mimicry. The controlled-carbohydrate approach, literally, mimics smoking, both chemically and psychologically.*

Chemical Mimicry

Let's return to chapter one for a moment to discuss this chemical mimicry. Two major biological events take place when you light up: 1.) a release in dopamine due to the activation of reward circuitry; 2.) a suppression of insulin secretion from the pancreas. I've got news for you: regarding the first of these two events, smoking is far from the only way to activate your reward circuitry.

Harken back to the days of Pavlov's salivating dog...what did he use as a reward? If you don't know, what do you give your dog when he doesn't pee on the rug? Not cigarettes, my friend...*food*.

That's right, food consumption is an even more effective, and natural, means of activating reward circuitry than nicotine! How does this fit into the Smoke Free Diet? *You can eat as much as you want...end of story*. When you crave a cigarette, eat. When you wake up, eat. When you go to bed, eat...eat in bed for all I care, *just as long as you eat the right foods*. Moreover, foods containing higher levels of protein and fat are far more hunger reducing than carb-filled foods, so you will likely end up eating less than you expect. But in the end, you can floss with string cheese for all I care...it doesn't matter because you can eat *as much as you want of the allowed foods without gaining a pound*; and again, this abundant food consumption activates the same biochemical feedback pathways as smoking. In the next chapter, you'll learn the implementation of the diet and its relationship to quitting, but you'll get one last week of nicotine hits. However, you'll very likely find that you crave less cigarettes even before you begin to taper off the smoking; again, this massive food intake mimics smoking at the neural level. The reason behind this is that very same concept I have drummed endlessly into your mind: nicotine releases dopamine in the reward circuitry; eating also releases dopamine in the reward circuitry, and at an even more primal level.

Let's move, now, to that other chemical event that takes place when you light up: the suppression of insulin release from the pancreas. We have talked about the ups and downs (hyper periods and crashes) of insulin spikes, but how does this relate to smoking? When you smoke, it calms you; one of the ways it does this, in addition to the release of dopamine, which can impart a sense of comfort, is by reducing insulin. As you learned in the first half of this chapter, the controlled-carbohydrate approach limits/eliminates insulin secretion from the pancreas, which eliminates insulin-induced mood swings; if you keep your insulin levels at a constant state of near-nothingness via proper eating, this mimics the effects of smoking on your pancreas. *So, in essence, simply by eating permitted foods in unlimited quantities, you have mimicked and replaced the two biological effects of smoking with natural and more potent replacements.*

Psychological Mimicry

So, we've discussed how the Smoke Free Diet will mimic the biological effects of smoking; how about the psychological aspects of addiction? Again, we come back to that wonderful concept: mimicry.

Let us revisit our list of "triggers" from chapter three.

Emotional
1. Stress reduction
2. Relaxation
3. Decreases boredom and/or loneliness
4. Feeling depressed when you don't (byproduct of dopamine reduction in the brain)
5. Alleviates anxiety

Situational

1. Comfortable distraction in social situations
2. Task-based; increases focus/concentration
3. Your friends are
4. After a meal
5. Morning ritual
6. Coffee or tea consumption
7. Alcohol consumption
8. Last thing you do before going to bed
9. Stops you from eating

Look over this list and count the number of triggers, emotional and/or situational, that could not be replaced by food; to top it off, number nine on the situational list might as well be erased from the metaphorical chalkboard.

Emotional Trigger Replacement

By substituting food for cigarettes, you're accomplishing a more powerful psychological task than simply replacing one item with another; you're mimicking the effects that cigarettes bring you. But this time, you're capitalizing upon the biological effects of the quantity-unrestricted Smoke Free Diet, as well.

The psychological addiction is born out of biology. There is a reason cigarettes decrease stress, cause relaxation, decrease boredom/loneliness, and alleviate depression and anxiety: dopamine release in the reward circuitry and the suppression of insulin release, the two biological effects of smoking, accomplish these tasks with great ease and efficiency. Remember that these two bodily substances are extremely powerful mood effectors. More dopamine in the brain and less insulin in the bloodstream will make you feel calm, focused, and relaxed. Moreover, a consistently elevated level of dopamine in the brain has been shown to exert an antidepressant and antianxiety ("anxiolytic") effect; in fact, some antidepressant and antianxiety medications rely on this same pathway, as does one of the most popular smoking-cessation prescription pills on the market, Zyban. So, logically, you can understand now why a sudden decrease in dopamine brought about by lowered nicotine levels results in a state of withdrawal that leads to depression and/or anxiety (and another pack of smokes). But once again, eating the Smoke Free way will eliminate these feelings by replacing them at the biological level, forever.

Situational Trigger Replacement

With the exception of increasing focus during tasks, which is a byproduct of elevated dopamine levels, situational triggers are the simple results of associations created by you and as such can be replaced just as easily by new associations. Look over the list of situational triggers again and try to imagine one situation that food could not serve as a replacement. Why can't you eat a low carb protein bar while out with friends, or snack on some nuts at the bar (which are carb-friendly in reasonable quantities, by the way)? When your friends light up, why can't you eat something to appease those salivary glands that fire up? As long as you avoid onions (which are carb friendly, by the way), your breath will smell a lot better than theirs, too. Instead of smoking after you eat, have a carb-friendly treat; there are enough carb-control candy bars on the market to fill the back seat of even the biggest sport-utility vehicle. When you wake up, eat instead of smoke, eat so much food that you can't even get up to smoke! Next time you have a cup of coffee, browse through the newly popular carb-controlled snacks available at nearly every coffeehouse; if you can't find one, bring one along, just in case. Alcohol? Well, as long as it's in sensible quantities and a carb-friendly liquor (and I don't even recommend that until you have officially quit and are advancing to the lifelong eating plan), again, enjoy! Nuts! Cheese! A steak! The options are limitless. I'll stop now to avoid being repetitive, but you can see that, just as in everyday life, associations are easily replaceable by new ones, and when you're done quitting, have reached your target weight, and have moved onto the lifelong eating phase, you'll still never have to worry about quantities again.

Chapter Five

Time to Waist Away and Kick Those Butts

Time to Start the Diet...Only

I do not recommend beginning the diet and quitting smoking on the same day, **period**. In fact, for reasons I am about to explain, you shouldn't even make both changes in the same week. However, there is one very narrow exception to this rule: if you are already, at the time of starting this program and for a period of greater than two weeks, eating in a controlled-carbohydrate manner at the level of restriction prescribed by the Smoke Free Diet (twenty grams of carbohydrates or less per day), you may begin the smoking-cessation program immediately.

In order to follow the Smoke Free Diet, you must watch what you eat. For those of you who have never done that, simply taking note of nutritional labels will be a jolt to the nervous system. You have to learn which foods are the right foods, you have to eat the right foods, and your body has to adapt to the diet.

That's right...unless you are eating in a controlled-carbohydrate manner at the level of restriction required by the Smoke Free Diet, your body will need a short period of adjustment. The reasoning is quite simple: your body has spent the last __ years using glucose (blood sugar) as its primary source of fuel, which means it has spent the last __ years with insulin floating around its blood vessels picking up all the fat you eat and routing it directly to your energy storage sites (i.e., your liver, muscles, stomach, and rear end).

As discussed in chapter four, *insulin has a powerful effect on mood*. Consider, again, the childhood sugar high. Insulin, when floating freely and in noteworthy concentrations about your blood plasma, can make you jumpy, hyper, anxious, and giddy, a state probably everybody has experienced at least once as a child; moreover, it always comes with its inevitable, logical opposite: the crash. This vacillating level of insulin can lead to, quite literally, an addiction to carbohydrates; books have been published on this very topic. A controlled-carbohydrate approach to eating eliminates such mood swings and rapid changes in energy levels; *once your body has switched over to its second most biologically available source of energy, stored fat, you will have an uninterrupted supply of energy without any accompanying crashes, period*. But, you must expect a short period of adjustment; it's like the end of a lifelong sugar-high.

But fear not; you're not going to turn into some monster. Your family is not going to put a contract on your head. You might feel a little tired for a couple days; then

again, you might not, as you have already prepared yourself for a lower level of insulin in the bloodstream simply by
smoking. However, just in case you do experience a little
fogginess in those first couple days, I recommend starting the diet on a weekend simply as a comfort measure.

Again, smoking may have prepared you for a controlled-carbohydrate lifestyle. How? As you now know,
nicotine use reduces insulin output from the pancreas,
and the Smoke Free Diet mimics this physiologic effect.
Therefore, by virtue of the fact that the average smoker
has less insulin output than the average nonsmoker, ***the
smoker may experience less withdrawal symptoms
from the reduction of insulin brought about by a
controlled-carbohydrate diet.*** In essence, again, you
have already prepared your body for a controlled carbohydrate lifestyle, just by smoking.

*But enough banter...unless, again, you are already
eating at the carbohydrate restriction level required by
this program, I suggest a week on the diet prior to ceas-
ing smoking.* But, good news: You'll be losing noticeable
weight within days...some people lose six to ten pounds in
this first two weeks!

Time to Quit

Now, once you have spent a week on the diet, a week
in which you should notice fat loss, more defined muscle
tone, less unpredictable surges of hunger, and an accompanying increase in energy, you'll be ready to begin the
smoking cessation portion of the program. However, keep
the following sentence in mind...stamp it on your forehead

if you have to: **you don't have to go cold turkey**. If you're feeling zealous, go for it, but I recommend gradual replacement over the period of a week. Once you know what to eat *and* that you can eat as much of it as you want, try replacing that morning cigarette with food. Then, try not to have that post-meal cigarette, and so on. Conquering even one ritual has powerful effects on the psyche; once you have proven to yourself and your subconscious that you can defeat embedded routines, deleting one more is easier than you think. Many people say that, if you can get past those initial few days of quitting, the rest is cake (just make sure it's carbohydrate-free cake).

Next, if you need or want to, you can use additional, assistive agents. The patch will help to quell the initial, physiologic cravings, but you need to flush the nicotine out of your system, so don't use it for longer than that first week; moreover, it does nothing for the psychological components. The gum and lozenges are helpful to some, but make sure they have no calories from carbohydrates (i.e., check the label for dextrose or any sugary ingredients). The gum and lozenges also assist with the oral fixation aspect of the addiction, but as you can eat as much as you want of all of these wonderful, satisfying foods, you will no doubt find the oral fixation easier to replace and conquer with food. There are some pill-form pharmacological agents that can offer assistance in quelling the withdrawal symptoms, as well; however, you should know that the primary mechanism of action of most of these pills is an increase in dopamine levels in the brain...the same mechanism as the Smoke Free Diet.

It's that simple. When you're craving a cigarette, eat a carbohydrate-free snack or meal. Eat as much of it as you want! You'll feel satisfied and rewarded, both chemically and psychologically. Remember, food activates reward circuitry in the brain and the lack of carbohydrates suppresses insulin output, thus producing that calming effect you previously got from cigarrettes. As we discussed at length in the last chapter, the mood-altering properties of cigarettes have been mimicked and replaced by food. So, eat, eat, and eat some more, as, provided you stick to the plan, you'll never have to worry about quantites again.

But What Do I Eat?

If you're anything like me, right now you're hoping I'll tell you exactly what to eat for the next month at every sitting. However, keep in mind that every smoker will experience different levels of cravings; some may not need to eat a ton of food, while some may require daily trips to the market. In that regard, giving you three meals a day to stick to would be an over generalization and a recipe for failure to those who require ten meals a day while quitting (and you'll still lose weight...can you believe that?). So, in that regard, I'll offer a general idea as to what to eat and, more importantly, what *not* to eat while on the Smoke Free Diet. Moreover, I will provide a list of some of my favorite carbohydrate-controlled recipes in the appendix, but keep in mind that there are literally thousands of recipes available on the Internet and in carb control cookbooks; just don't forget to check the carb counts and pay attention to serving sizes.

Typical carbohydrate-controlled diets say to limit your carbohydrate consumption to anywhere between twenty to forty grams per day in order to lose weight. I say: shoot for zero, but make sure you don't go over twenty during the initial week. The closer you get to zero carbohydrates, the less blood sugar your body has to feed from and the less insulin you will produce; consequently, the biological switch from using blood sugar for energy to stored fat will happen more quickly. However, as eating zero carbohydrates is nearly impossible (even meat can have a couple of grams), this is more of a worthy goal than an iron-clad rule; we shoot for zero and accept twenty or under for the first week. After the first week, forty carbs or less per day is acceptable until you've comfortably quit smoking. After you've quit and reached your target weight, you can advance to the lifelong eating plan for the addictive personality, described later.

   -**Week 1**: Consume twenty grams of carbohydrates or less per day spread as evenly as possible across all meals
   -**Week 2 and until you've comfortably quit, as well as reached your target weight**: Consume forty grams or less of carbohydrates per day spread as evenly as possible across all meals
   -**Reached target weight**: Lifelong eating plan (follows in chapter six)

OK, Already...The Food!
   During the quitting phase, the time until you complete the smoking cessation portion of the program, limit your

dietary intake to unrestricted quantities (expect where noted along with specific carb counts of those foods) of the following foods. Be cognizant and wary of additives and/or condiments, such as in pre-marinated chicken and fish.

All Fish

Tuna, Salmon, Sole, Trout, Flounder, Sardines, Herring, Anchovies

All Meat

Beef, Pork, Lamb, Veal, Venison, Ham*, Bacon*

*Processed meats, such as ham, bacon, pepperoni, salami, hot dogs ,and other luncheon meats may have added sugar and thus contribute hidden carbohydrates.

All Fowl

Chicken, Turkey, Duck, Goose, Cornish Hen, Quail, Pheasant

All Shellfish

Oysters, Crabmeat, Shrimp, Lobster, Clams, Squid, Mussels

All Eggs

Scrambled, Fried, Poached, Deviled, Hard-boiled, Soft-boiled, Omelets

Cheeses

Cheddar, Cream Cheese, Swiss, Mozzarella, Gouda, Goat, Roquefort, Other Blue Cheeses

Low-carbohydrate Vegetables

Peppers, Mushrooms, Celery, Cucumber, Lettuce, Romaine Lettuce, Radishes, Bok Choy, Parsley, Artichoke, Asparagus, Spinach, Broccoli, Cherry Tomatoes, Cabbage, Cauliflower, Zucchini

Salad Garnishes

Grated Cheese, Sour Cream, Hard-boiled Egg, Mushrooms, Bacon, Oil, Vinegar, Full-fat Salad Dressing

All Herbs & Spices

Garlic, Basil, Pepper, Dill, Thyme, Oregano, Ginger, Rosemary, Sage

Fats and Oils

Olive Oil, Vegetable Oil, Canola Oil, Walnut Oil, Soybean Oil, Grapeseed Oil, Sesame Oil, Sunflower Oil, Safflower Oil, Butter

Beverages

Filtered, Mineral, Spring, Tap Water, Club Soda, Heavy Cream, Decaf Coffee, Decaf Tea, Herb Tea, Lemon Juice, Diet Beverages (Count each artificially sweetened-beverage as one gm/carbs.)

Low/Moderate Carbohydrate Vegetables (Some Moderation Required; Check Carb Counts Below)

Broccoli (4 gram carbs per 3.5 oz), Spaghetti Squash (10 gram carbs per cup), Eggplant (6 gram carbs per 3.5 oz), Brussels Sprouts (6 gram carbs per 3.5 oz), Tomato

(Small-5 gram carbs; Medium-7 gram carbs; Large-12 gram carbs), Turnips (3 gram carbs per 3.5 oz), Onion (9 gram carbs per 3.5 oz)

Artificial Sweeteners (Some Moderation Required; Count Each Packet as One Gram Carb)
Sucralose (Splenda), Saccharin (Sweet N' Low), NutraSweet (Equal)

Carbohydrate-controlled Snacks and Pre-made Foods
A practically unlimited variety of carbohydrate-controlled snacks and foods exist in nearly every grocery and convenience store. Take advantage of them; some of them are nearly identical in taste to their carbohydrate-uncontrolled counterparts. Make sure to check the "net carbohydrate" count and add *that* number to your daily total. *If the net carb count is not offered, subtract grams of fiber and grams of sugar alcohols (sometimes noted as "other carbs") from the total carbs, and you will have computed your net carb count.*
Worthy of note: many controlled-carbohydrate snacks, especially those of the sweet variety (protein bars and ice creams, for example), incorporate engineered sweetening techniques and chemicals that claim not to raise blood sugar. One example of such a chemical used in this manner is malitol. According to manufacturers, grams of malitol do not raise blood sugar in a manner significant enough to count as a "net" carbohydrate; instead, it is counted as an "other carbohydrate," or more technically

a "sugar alcohol." These do not count toward net, or "countable" carbohydrates. While this is fine and dandy, and you are permitted to count only the net carbs toward your daily total, heed my words regarding sugar alcohols: the body has an average threshold for sugar alcohols of twenty grams per day. If you exceed this amount, you may experience indigestion, gas, and/or diarrhea. Of course, this varies from person to person, but this is the average, so why take the chance? Use these snacks sparingly; consider them supplements designed and intended to curb the occasional sweet tooth.

Chapter Six

Dietary Supplements

Dietary supplements can be a blessing or a curse, depending upon which ones you take and your knowledge of the ingredients. The following section lists everything from highly recommended supplements to the dangerous, avoid-at-all-cost ones; please read it very carefully before tearing off to the vitamin store. Also, take a moment to consider the following definition of "dietary supplement" from a very reputable dictionary: "a product taken orally that contains one or more ingredients that are intended to suppement one's diet and are not considered food." Read that carefully, multiple times if you have to...supplements are not replacements, but additives to an eating regimen. If you choose to employ dietary supplements, an example being protein-based shakes, do not use them in lieu of food, as this could result in deficiencies *caused* by supplements, which is counter to their defined purpose.

Multivitamins

Everybody should be taking a multivitamin, not just people on special diets or quitting smoking. But as you may have noticed walking down the aisle at your local drug store, there are quite a few multis on the market. It seems as if vitamin manufacturers have concocted a formula for every demographic: man, woman, overweight, athletic, elderly, young, active, inactive, and every combination of the above. There's even a new market for people on low-carbohydrate diets; these vitamins boast a potent B complex collection, as well as biotin, a mineral that, supposedly, assists in the breakdown of fat.

In truth, you can just find the one that fits you best and take it, but I have tried nearly all of them and find a more unconventional type to work best. In the same aisle, you'll find (probably on the bottom shelf for size purposes) boxes of multivitamin "packets." Each packet has multiple, individual pills, representing nearly every class of vitamin and mineral in singular form. The vitamin C is one pill; the vitamin E is another. These packet multis almost always contain high doses of the essentials and still come in types for every demographic. I take the "stress complex" variety, as this usually implies higher levels of B complex vitamins, which are good for energy levels and muscle tissue repair. All in all, regardless of which, just make sure you're taking a multivitamin...and that it isn't sweetened with sugar (check those carb counts!).

Fiber Supplements

I recommend a carbohydrate-free fiber supplement, such as psyllium husk, to ward off possible constipation due to the increased protein intake and, depending upon your choice of foods, decreased fiber intake. You may also choose to incorporate a homeopathic cleanse in lieu of the fiber supplement periodically; these products cleanse your entire system, from your skin to your colon, but vary in length of program time (anywhere from one week to one month, depending upon directions and personal needs). If you choose to use a cleanser, I recommend "Dfense" by Wellness Pro or "Ultimate Cleanse" by Nature's Secret; these particular cleansing programs are lengthy enough to last through the quitting regimen and will more than get your system "moving." You should not use a cleansing system and a fiber supplement at the same time; most cleansing systems have sufficient fiber already. Also, note that homeopathic cleansing should be limited to no more than twice per year and for no more than one month each time, as more than this can create a systemic addiction and actually increase the likelihood of constipation.

Niacin:

Did you know that niacin (vitamin B3) was once called nicotinic acid? Sound similar to anything? Research suggests that niacin is so similar to nicotine that it binds to the same receptors in your brain. These receptors start to feel a deficiency when you quit smoking, or even cut down; this healthy alternative may fool them into thinking you haven't. Niacin is also known to assist the circulatory system; given the additional stress smoking has placed on your heart and blood vessels, this is a wonderful bonus. Niacin should be a part of your morning regimen during this program and for at least a period of a few months after completely quitting to help prevent relapse. Make sure you buy the "flush-free" variety, as niacin can cause an itchy sensation unless it is time-released. My personal favorite is available at nearly every major drug-store: Nature's Bounty Flush-Free Niacin (500mg).

Fat Burners

I will preface this section by telling you that I have spent many years studying biochemistry and pharmacology. Moreover, the most significant portion of this time, and the most important discoveries I have made during these academic pursuits, relate directly to the subject matter of this section: stimulant drugs. In other words... take the information I am about to impart very seriously. I will also preface this section by giving due credit to the sports supplement industry; the geniuses that brought you over-the-counter, fat-burning supplements have spent years discovering and exploiting governmental, chemical, and marketing loopholes that have made them billions of dollars, but at what cost?

Almost everybody heard about the ephedrine scandal, the one that led to us having to swipe our ID's at pharmacy counters for cold medicine. Famous sports stars and kids alike were dying on the playing field, their veins pumped full of legal and widely available supplements touting "increased energy" and "fat-burning" potential. The big question seemed to be this: How did the Food and Drug Administration let something like this end up on the shelves of nearly every retail store in town, from gas stations to supermarkets? The answer to this question may shock you: the FDA doesn't regulate all such products because the supplement manufacturers have found a loophole.

Getting any standard drug, from Tylenol to prescription painkillers, on the market is a multi-year, multimillion-dollar process regulated carefully and with great scrutiny by the Food and Drug Administration. Every drug is, almost invariably, born in an animal research laboratory and over the course of years undergoes millions of dollars' worth of clinical trials in multiple and progressively more advanced animal species, finally reaching humans. Had the ephedrine-containing, fat-burning supplements undergone the standard drug protocol, chances are high that they would not have made it to the market; but they were not subject to such a scrutinizing test period. Why? The answer to this question may shock you, as well: supplement industry ephedrine, the kind found in vitamin isle "fat-burners," is imported into this country in plant form as an herb called "ma huang." The Food and Drug Administration has no jurisdiction over the importation and exportation of plant-based anything; the Department of Agriculture does. Unfortunately, ma huang importation and use was not a file drawer at the FDA until people started noticing complications stemming from its use. A few years later, ephedrine-containing products were removed from the market, and the nutrition supplement industry lost its golden goose—but not for long. As I said, these people are, truly, geniuses. Instead of crying over losing ephedrine, they capitalized upon it in a seemingly responsible and borderline apologetic manner, marketing new, equally effective, "ephidrine-free" alternatives, with nearly identical and equally dangerous active ingredients.

"Ephedrine free" does not mean that your heart and endocrine system will not be under full-scale attack. You see, all the supplement industry needed was a similar compound to ephedrine that could be imported in plant form. The first one they jumped on was/is called bitter orange extract, which has an active chemical component called synephrine. Synephrine has been called the "kissing cousin" of ephedrine, and operates in nearly an identical manner. First, they both are potent vasoconstrictors, meaning that they cause your blood vessels to constrict and your heart to work harder, which burns more calories. But this can lead to such nasty side effects as high blood pressure, enlarged heart muscle, and in the case of existing health problems (such as high cholesterol or blood pressure), the possibility of stroke or cardiac arrest. Second, they increase the production and circulation of adrenaline in your system. Adrenaline increases heart rate and respiration; combine this with blood vessels that are narrower from smoking, and you have a cardiovascular system that may choose to give up rather than work under such conditions. Also, when your adrenal glands (the adrenaline factories) are stimulated to produce extra adrenaline by such chemicals, they may end up producing less naturally (without pills in your system), which can lead to fatigue and a resulting state of addiction.

There are a couple more tricks that the supplement gurus have employed, and these tricks even enable them to market their products as "stimulant free" and/or "all natural." In truth, the statements "stimulant free" and "all natural" are true, but only in the sense that the pills themselves don't have potent stimulants embedded in them. Instead, they activate your body's naturally occurring stimulants but at unhealthy levels. One means for accomplishing such a task is a potent dose of L-tyrosine, a naturally occurring amino acid that your body uses to produce the four "monoamines," or the primary neurotransmitters: dopamine, seratonin, norepinephrine, and epinephrine (adrenaline). Those little shots of energy sold at gas stations and advertised all over TV are "all-naturally" filled to the brim with L-tyrosine. In small doses, L-tyrosine is relatively benign and can even give your mood a little boost without leading to dependence or addiction. However, the supplement companies are packing these pills and drinks with unbelievable amounts of L-tyrosine, which causes your body to produce an excess of monoamines, especially epinephrine (adrenaline). Hark...we're back at the same place that ephedrine and synephrine brought us: elevated heart rate, blood pressure, and respiration. Moreover, since L-tyrosine is necessary for production of the monoamines, taking too much in pill form can lead to dependence and a long-term reduction of monoamine production, including a deficit in dopamine, which will make you crave cigarettes. Monoamine deficits have also been linked to other mood disorders, primarily depression. Watch out for this clever trick in "energy drinks" sold everywhere.

One more trick that took me a few hours of staring at labels to figure out is the thyroid trick; this trick is how that former exotic dancer gone reality-TV star lost weight so quickly before tragically dying of an overdose. Your thyroid gland and the thyroid hormone it produces are responsible for regulation of your metabolism. Too little thyroid hormone will slow your metabolism down; too much and you may find yourself jittery, sweating, and anxious...but, you will be thin. One naturally occurring chemical that causes an increase in thyroid hormone secretion is iodine. Some supplement companies are pumping their products full of iodine in an effort to increase thyroid hormone output and thus artificially raise your metabolism (and heart rate, blood pressure, respiration, anxiety levels...). Extended use will lead to, you guessed it: dependence. Watch out for fat burners that warn you not to take them if you are allergic to shellfish; as shellfish contain large amounts of iodine, this is code for "don't take me."

So, what does all this boil down to? **Don't take fat burners.** They're dangerous, especially for smokers, and even more for smokers who are not at their target weights. Smoking causes vasoconstriction (narrowing of blood vessels) that, over years, can become somewhat constant; by quitting smoking, you will give your body a chance to repair this damage and your heart will no longer be working as hard. If you're an overweight smoker, there is a possibility that your cholesterol and blood pressure are already elevated, which means your heart is under some additional stress. The good news is that by following the Smoke Free Diet, you will lower these vitals very quickly, but adding fat burners to the mix creates a very, very dangerous combination.

Protein Powders

Protein powders are very good *supplements* to typical American diets, especially in the case of resistance-training athletes. Proteins are, after all, the building blocks of muscle; without it, you cannot add tone or strength, and if you resistance train without adequate protein intake, it can actually lead to muscle loss rather than gain. But do you need to supplement protein consumption while on the Smoke Free Diet? That depends. If you eat a high-protein combination (meat-heavy, for example) of the allowed foods, then, no, you don't. Chances are high that you will garner more than enough protein from the diet to support muscle gain and prevent any loss if you choose to resistance train. If you find yourself concentrating more on the vegetables than the protein, then go ahead and buy a can of protein powder (again, I'm a big fan of Wellness Pro products, as they are low in carbs, as well as more grounded in medical and athletic research than any company I've come across in seventeen years of resistance training). However, whichever brand you choose, make sure it's carbohydrate controlled and that you either mix it with water or another low carbohydrate base.

Timing is also important when supplementing with protein. It is highly recommended that you consume protein after a workout to optimize the post-training "window of opportunity," the time when your muscles are highly sensitive to protein intake due to the damage incurred during the workout. Also, these protein powders can produce a calming effect, as they typically have naturally occurring L-tryptophan (that stuff in turkey that puts you to sleep on Thanksgiving) but not enough that if you use them during the day, you'll find yourself drowsy. Again, use is a matter of personal choice, rather than need; personally, I love a good smoothie now and again.

Amino Acids

Proteins are the building blocks of muscle, but amino acids are the building blocks of protein. So, by the transitive property, if you're getting an adequate supply of protein from your diet, they are not necessary. For those of you not getting a high level of protein, choose the protein powder over the amino acids. Each scoop of protein tends to have an exponentially higher allotment of amino acids (you can almost always find the profiles on the side of the jugs) than you can buy in pill form, and the powder is much, much cheaper.

Creatine

I do not recommend the use of supplemental creatine for multiple reasons. First, it is unnecessary if consuming high levels of meat, as meat is our natural source of creatine. Second, supplemental creatine may increase muscle size, but it is somewhat of a façade. Creatine acts as a super hydrator of sorts, allowing your muscles to soak up water like balloons; but the only way you can maintain this increased muscle tone is by using supplemental creatine constantly, and this has been linked with some possible side effects, like hair loss and indigestion. All in all, save your money on the creatine. If you want muscle, follow an exercise routine consistently and eat the appropriate foods; you will build it yourself.

Essential Fatty Acids

EFAs, as they're popularly called, are wonder supplements for decreasing inflammation and cholesterol, as well as for mood regulation and increasing lean muscle mass, but only if you're not getting enough in your diet already. Diets high in fat, such as the one you are following, are chock-full of EFAs, *especially* if you eat lots of fish (so pile on the salmon). Like the powders and amino acids, I only recommend EFAs if you are not eating high levels of protein.

Chapter Seven

A Lifelong Eating Plan for the Addictive Personality

So, you've quit smoking. How good does it feel? You've taken a step that will add years to your life and exponentially increase the quality of those years as well. You've increased the likelihood that you'll meet your grandchildren...maybe even your great grandchildren. You've chosen freedom over enslavement, and those who love you will thank you for it when you're standing by their sides for years to come.

If you've also reached your target weight during the quitting portion of the program, it is time to move on to the lifelong eating plan; if you have not, continue on the eating plan until you are at the weight you wish to achieve, then move on to the lifelong plan, below.

The Lifelong Plan

The lifelong eating plan still does not restrict quantity, but it does require some initial research into your own metabolism. After this, expect and enjoy a lifetime of gluttonous eating, immeasurable energy, and stable weight.

The first thing you need to do is pick a day to begin the lifelong plan; I recommend a Monday for ease. Very simply, weigh yourself that Monday morning (before eating or drinking anything); then, during that first week, increase your carbohydrate intake by ten grams per day (so, if you were eating forty grams per day, increase to fifty per day). Then, on Sunday, at the same time and under the same circumstances, weigh yourself. If you are still losing weight, simply add another ten grams per day (for this example, increase to sixty grams per day) of carbohydrates for the following week.

Repeat this weekly routine until you find your "sweet spot," or that carbohydrate quantity that allows you to maintain your target weight without losing or gaining. Remember, you're still not counting calories, only carbohydrates, and you can still eat all the carb-free, fat-full foods you have been enjoying all along.

If you find that during the first week of the maintenance plan you gain a pound or two after increasing your daily intake by ten grams of carbs, fear not; just subtract ten grams of daily carbs the following week, which will put you back in fat burn mode and the weight will fall right off. The week after that, add five grams instead of the ten you added last time. It is nearly certain that this five-gram increase, rather than the ten that caused some weight gain, will be your "sweet spot." This type of extreme sensitivity almost never occurs, so take the time to evaluate your eating pattern over the week in question.

Did you consume all of your carbs in one sitting on one or more days? Did you go over your intended intake without meaning to? Were your carbs coming from mostly high-glycemic index food sources (i.e., candy, potato chips, etc.)? Did you check those nutrition labels? *Any of these mistakes can sabotage the lifelong plan.*

This lifelong plan allows you to eat as much as you want for, as it implies, *life*. During this transition, you can begin to add back some of the foods you may have missed during the quitting phase: nuts, berries, a small bowl of lower-carb cereal in the morning, maybe even some whole-grain, high-fiber bread here and there (check those carb counts, though). You're still not counting calories or quantities, only carbohydrates. You're maintaining your weight now, instead of losing, because you've found a weight at which you're comfortable, and that makes you feel good about yourself. If you ever binge for a week (somebody force-feeds you a bag of french fries every day, for example) and you gain a pound or two, just cut back the following week by ten grams of carbs, even twenty if you're in a hurry, and it'll fall right back off. You see, in addition to the freedom you have gained by giving up smoking, you've discovered a lifelong plan for weight maintenance that allows you the freedom to change and update your weight whenever you feel like it...and freedom, my friend, is the greatest gift of all.

Chapter Eight

Exercise: Fit from the Inside-Out

Should you choose (notice, I said "choose") to incorporate exercise into your lifestyle, you will not regret it. In the context of smoking cessation, exercise releases even more of those "reward chemicals" into your system (ever heard of the runner's high?), again mimicking the biochemical effects of smoking. In the context of weight loss, exercise will dramatically expedite the effects of the Smoke Free Diet.

There are, primarily, two types of exercise: aerobic (think running or cycling) and anaerobic (think weightlifting). Aerobic exercise increases the body's need for oxygen, causing an elevation in pulse rate and calorie expenditure during the session. Anaerobic exercise increases lean muscle mass, as well as burns calories both during the session *and* for extended periods following the session. The reasoning behind this anaerobic "afterburn" is threefold:

1. While the movements are shorter in duration, they are, still, physically exerting, and, thus, require calories to perform.
2. Anaerobic exercise, such as weightlifting, literally damages muscle fibers, forcing the body to rebuild itself following each workout. The reason you gain muscle tone from this damage is an evolutionary adaptation to stress: your muscles will increase in size and strength to avoid sustaining similar damage in the future. This rebuilding process requires calories and continues for hours, even days, after your workout.
3. Increasing lean muscle mass elevates your basal metabolic rate, as muscle tissue requires heightened levels of calories to sustain its existence. *The more muscle you have, the more calories you burn at rest.*

If you plan to begin an exercise program and have not performed any physical fitness activities in a significant amount of time, **start slow!** A good rule of thumb for aerobic exercise intensity is that you should be able to have a conversation while you're performing it, but not to sing a song; in seventeen years of avid fitness, I have never come across an easier or more effective technique for reaching and maintaining your target heart rate (the rate that places you square in the fat-burning zone without sacrificing muscle in the process). Start at no more than thirty minutes of aerobic exercise every other day, only increasing the duration and/or intensity when completely comfortable; if you choose to perform aerobic and anaerobic exercise, it is perfectly acceptable to do them on the same day. Just take note, before you excitedly increase your durations on the stairmaster or stationary bike, excessive aerobic exercise can sacrifice muscle tone (picture running or biking through a forest for endless periods of time...your body will, naturally, seek to shed the heaviest baggage, which is muscle over fat *by a long shot*), and muscle burns calories just existing. Competitive physique models usually don't go more than forty-five minutes on an aerobic machine because they, or their trainers, are aware of this lesser-known tidbit.

I highly recommend everybody perform anaerobic exercise, such as weightlifting, as the more muscle you have on your body, the higher your basal metabolic rate will be (the calories you burn just existing). Moreover, as we age, our bones become more brittle; bearing wieght has been shown to combat this powerfully. If you wish, you can utilize Web sites such as www.bodybuilding.com or online databases from fitness magazines to find beginner routines; there are hundreds of routines for every style of lifter, from beginner to advanced, woman or man, all the way to competitive level all over the Internet. The single most important variable, however, is consistency. To give you a good starting point, I would recommend three days per week of lifting, targeting all the major muscle groups in each session with three working sets and eight to twelve repetitions (reps) per set. When I say eight to twelve reps per set, I mean that you should use a weight that provides enough resistance to make you tired somewhere between eight to twelve reps. These exercises will be performed using the most basic and universally available machines, or with standard dumbbells if you prefer for the bicep curls...a five-minute tour of the gym will more than suffice for locating them.

If you have read the detailed exercise descriptions that follow the routine below, studied the illustrations, and still feel uncomfortable getting acquainted with the movements, do not despair....the gym staff is always happy to show you proper technique, hands-on.

Example:

Machine Chest Press: 3 sets of 8-12 reps

Machine Shoulder Press: 3 sets of 8-12 reps

Assisted Pull-up: 3 sets of 8-12 reps

Leg Press: 3 sets of 8-12 reps

Bicep Curls: 3 sets of 8-12 reps

Tricep Pressdowns: 3 sets of 8-12 reps

Machine Chest Press

Locate the machine and, if adjustable, assure that the pressing handles are at a comfortable starting distance in front of your body and at mid-chest; you want a slight stretch without inciting any discomfort, especially if you have any shoulder or rotator cuff injuries. Usually, about six inches away from the sternum is a good starting point. Choose a weight that you can lift eight to twelve times; you want to feel fatigued at the end of the "set," as if you could not muster any additional repetitions. Perform three sets of eight to twelve reps.

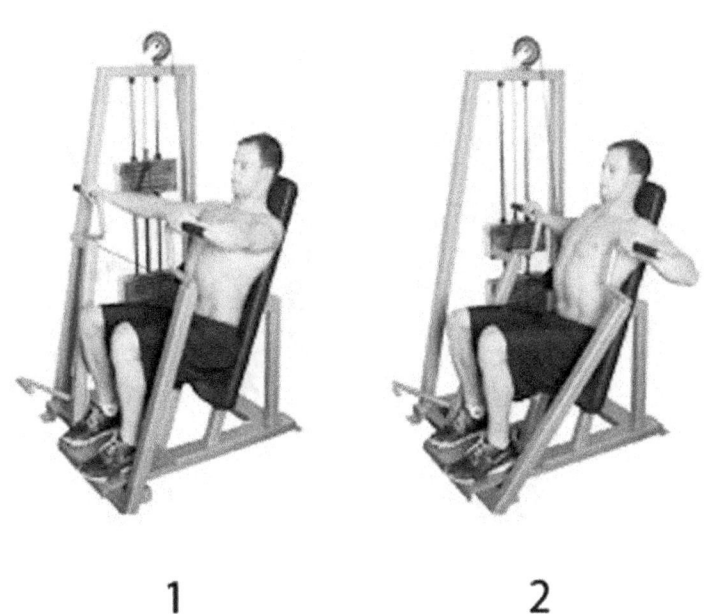

1   2

Machine Shoulder Press

Sit in machine and adjust handles to a comfortable starting position directly above shoulder height; if width is adjustable, you want your hands three to four inches away from the outermost point of the shoulder. Again, choose a weight that you can lift eight to twelve times but that fatigues you by the final rep, and perform three sets.

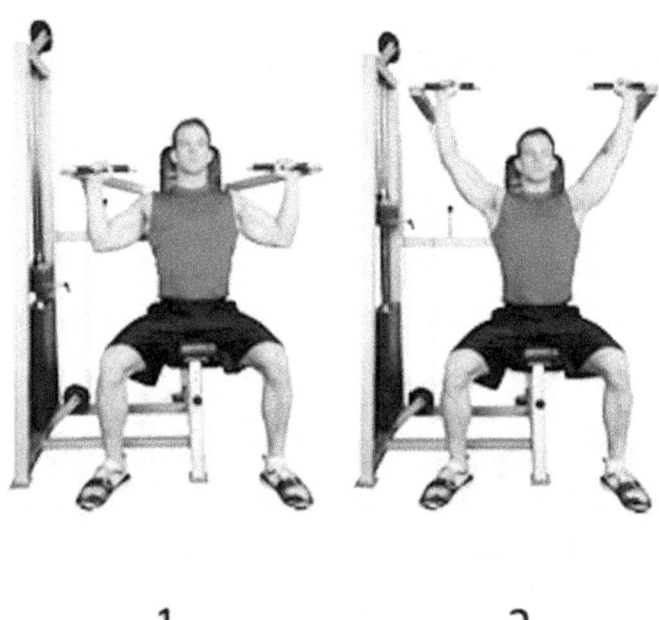

1   2

Assisted Pull-up

Nearly every gym in the world has assisted pull-up machines. First locate the machine, which should have steps to enter and a bar to place your knees or feet on for assistance, as well as the requisite pull-up handles above. Experiment to find an assistive weight to counter your own body weight that allows you to complete the same eight to twelve reps. Keeping your body vertical and your eyes pointed forward, grasp whichever handles are the most comfortable (palms together, forward, or toward you) and perform eight to twelve reps for three sets.

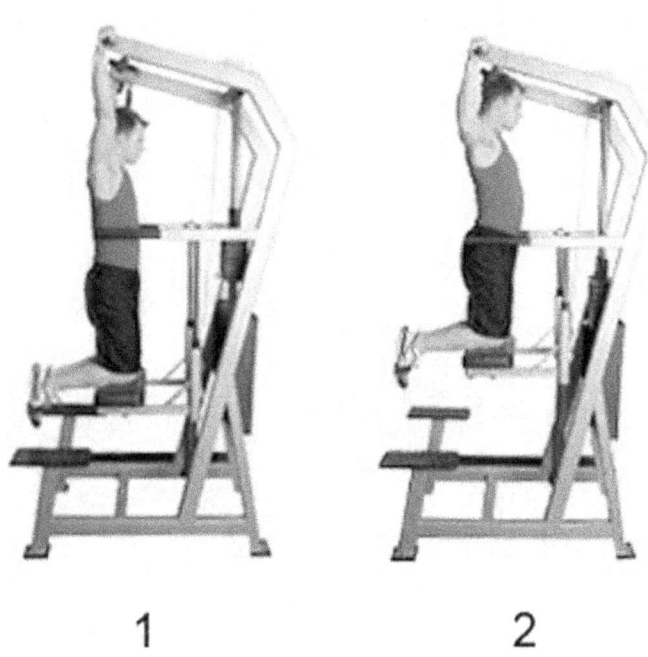

1   2

Leg Press Machine

Sit in machine and place feet on pad approximately shoulder width apart. Adjust starting point of feet (or bend in knee) to a comfortable distance so that at your starting point you are not rounding your lower back, but not so far away that the movement is only a few inches once you start pushing. For safety measures, on machines that require you to physically place the weight plates onto the machine (see illustration), start with no weight and add small increments to each side until you reach a weight that is suitable and comfortable for eight to twelve reps and three sets. If your gym offers a machine version with a moveable pin for weight levels, this is a safer option and the same instructions apply minus the need to physically add or remove weight plates. Simply move the pin up or down until you find the weight that fatigues you at 8-12 reps.

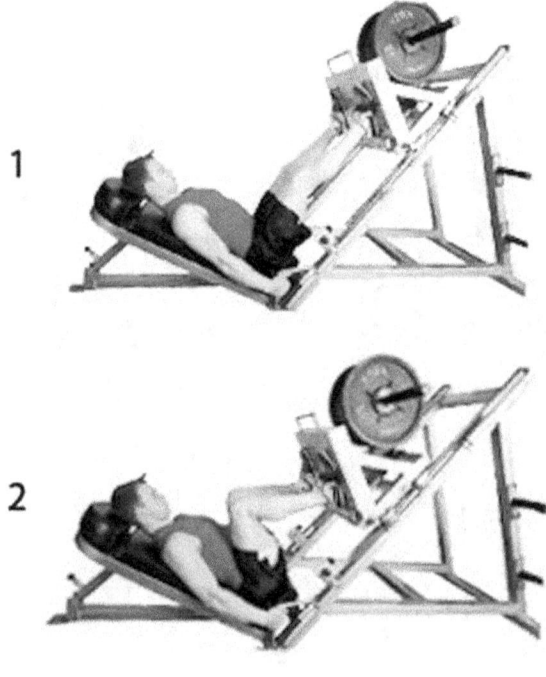

Bicep Curl

This exercise can be performed on a machine, with free floating dumbbells while seated, or standing with a weighted bar; whichever you choose, the concept remains the same. You will be isolating your biceps by elevating and lowering the weight using the elbow as the "hinge." In fact, the movement takes place only at the elbow; the rest of your body should remain as immobile as possible to avoid cheating and/or back injuries. If you're standing, don't swing your arms for momentum...keep your elbows locked at your side. If you're seated, keeping your back firmly against the pad helps to prevent the same mistake. I will place illustrations below of the dumbbell variation, which can also be performed seated; the same three sets of eight to twelve reps applies.

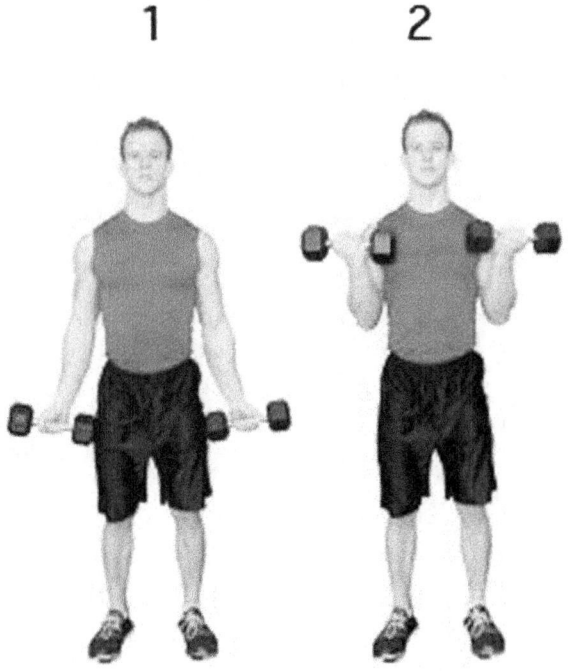

1   2

Tricep Pressdown

Locate a cable/pulley machine and choose the attachment that looks like a triangular rope (the most popular attachment). Attach it to the upper pulley and stand facing the machine. Grasp the ends of the rope with palms facing toward each other in front of you, then pull the rope down until your arms are tucked at your side with your elbows still bent. This is your starting position. You want to keep your elbows locked against your midsection for the entire movement; like the bicep movement, the hinge point is your elbow and this isolates the triceps. Slowly press the rope straight down using your triceps and, upon reaching a point near which your elbows are locked straight out, *slowly* push the rope ends outward across your body as if you're attempting to spread the triangle into a straight line. The movement starts with your palms facing toward each other and ends with them facing downward (see illustration). Experiment to find your eight to twelve rep weight and perform three sets of 8-12.

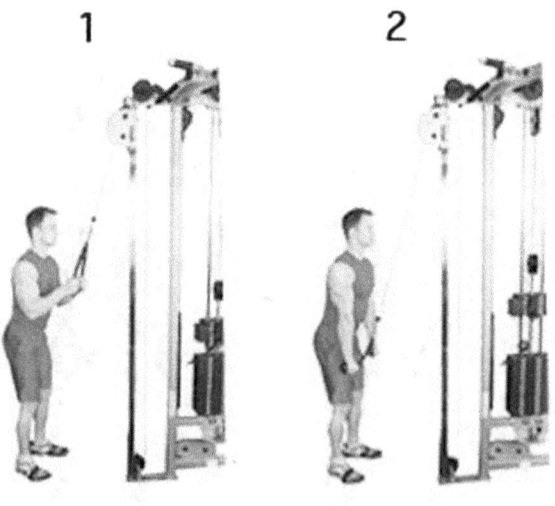

1   2

Chapter Nine

Final Tips to Beef Up Your Arsenal

The Training Partner

Chances are very high that you know somebody who smokes; chances are also high that you know somebody who smokes that would like to quit, even if he/she has not voiced the desire. If you have knowledge that a smoker you know would like to quit, why not suggest a partnership? Quit smoking together, lose weight together, and get in the best shape of your life...together! It's nice to have a support system in any task. If you know somebody who smokes, or many people who smoke, but don't know that he/she/they would like to quit, why not casually mention that you're going to try this method? Don't forget to mention all of the added bonuses (weight reduction, vitals reduction, gluttonous eating privileges). If he/she/they have not heard of the Smoke Free Diet, belief levels may be low, so it may be smart to have a copy of your book handy or a good speech written on index cards in your pocket.

If you don't know somebody who smokes, or if you do but prefer not to ask him/her/them, chances are probably high that you know somebody who wishes *you* didn't smoke, like a significant other or child. These types of training partners can be the best support systems of all, as there is that little, added bonus of their having a vested interest in your health and lifespan. Moreover, even if the partner is a nonsmoker, he/she can join you on your dietary quest. If your nonsmoking partner is already at a comfortable weight but still wishes to join you for whatever reason, be it support, curiosity, or an interest in eating until he/she can't stand up straight without gaining any body fat...wonderful! If the training partner is a live-in, you can even share the cooking and shopping duties.

Finally, and I'm covering every possible hypothetical I can think of, if the theoretical training partner is a supportive nonsmoker, but does not wish to embark on the low-carbohydrate lifestyle and prefers the couch to the gym, at least you can have somebody to call when you need a little moral support; sometimes, just a nudge from somebody who cares can go a long way.

Letting Your Smoking Buddies Know

Assuming you hang around people who smoke and you can't convince every one of them to quit, it is highly advisable to let them know you are quitting. Quitting is becoming increasingly socially acceptable as smoking becomes increasingly unacceptable. If they know you're quitting, they're more likely to refrain from lighting up in front of you, and if they don't exercise that courtesy, they will understand when you choose to either leave the clouded scene or whip out a carb-free protein bar when they do light up. Be sure to have breath mints ready for them, or nose plugs for yourself, as you're going to realize very soon how bad you once smelled.

Keep Food Close at Hand

I recommend that you plan ahead for cravings. Heck... go to the army surplus store, buy some of those cargo pants with lots of pockets, and stuff them full of carb-free snacks. Or if you don't feel like doing that for fashion or convenience reasons, keep some in your car, desk, and of course your refrigerator. Stock up when you go to the market, at least for a couple of days at a time; that way, if a craving strikes at an odd time, you won't need to screech off to the gas station for a low-carb snack in your pajamas.

Time for the Supermarket

You now have the "know-how" and the "know-why" to begin this journey, so grab that acceptable food list and go to the supermarket. You understand now that the Smoke Free Diet will liberate you from the bonds of smoking, as well as provide a lifelong eating plan to keep you healthy, inside and out. So, eat, eat, and eat some more...because, as an esteemed cardiologist, biochemist, and ardent supporter of my program once said: "String cheese has never been linked to lung cancer."

Appendix A: Easy and Savory Low-carb Recipes

Obviously, an exhaustive list of all available low-carbohydate recipes would take another volume of books, so I am choosing from among my favorites to give you a sample, as well as an implied arsenal of ingredients by virtue of their inclusion in the recipes. Try a few; you will quickly learn that this manner of eating need not be tasteless. In fact, I think you'll agree with most followers of this dietary lifestyle that eating according to the Smoke Free Diet feels more like an exercise in gluttony than a diet.

Blackened Salmon

Nutritional Information Per Serving
Net Carbs: 1 gram
Fiber: 1 gram
Protein: 35 grams
Fat: 37 grams
Calories: 490

Recipe Information
Makes: 4 servings
Prep Time: 0:14:00
Marinate Time: N/A
Cook Time: 0:6:00

Cool Time: N/A

Ingredients

1 tablespoon dried thyme

1 tablespoon dried oregano

1 tablespoon Old Bay seasoning*

1 teaspoon salt

1 teaspoon ground black pepper

4 (6-ounce) salmon steaks, ½-inch thick

¼ cup canola oil, divided

Directions

Combine the thyme, oregano, Old Bay seasoning, salt, and pepper in a small bowl. Coat each salmon steak with 2 teaspoons of oil; press seasoned rub into flesh on both sides. Heat the remaining 4 teaspoons oil in a large cast-iron skillet over medium-high heat. Add the salmon and sear until coating is black, about 3 minutes per side. Serve right away with low-carbohydrate vegetables such as broccoli or spinach, and top off with a low-carb dessert.

*A combination of herbs and spices, including celery seed, mustard, red pepper, black pepper, bay leaf, cloves, allspice, ginger, mace, cardamom, cinnamon, paprika, and salt, Old Bay seasoning is great for seafood dishes and works on almost all other savory dishes. You can find it in the spice and herb aisle of any supermarket.

Asian Vegetable Bowl

Nutritional Information Per Serving:

Net Carbs: 6.0 grams

Fiber: 1.5 grams
Protein: 6.5 grams
Fat: 2.5 grams
Calories: 74

Recipe Information:
Makes: 6 servings
Prep Time: 0:10:00
Marinate Time: N/A
Cook Time: 0:10:00
Cool Time: N/A

Ingredients
6 cups reduced-sodium chicken broth
4 tablespoons lite (reduced-sodium) soy sauce
2 cups bok choy, sliced (Chinese cabbage; use half leaves and
half stems)
4 ounces exotic mixed sliced mushrooms (about 2 cups)
1 tablespoon fresh ginger, sliced or grated
1 garlic clove, very thinly sliced
1 Thai or Serrano chili, seeded and minced
1 cup diced tomatoes
3 green onions, sliced (about ½ cup)
6 ounces soft or firm tofu, cut into ½ inch dice
1 medium carrot, peeled and shredded (about ½ cup)
1½ tablespoons fresh cilantro, chopped

Directions
In a large saucepan, bring broth and soy sauce to a boil.
Reduce heat; add bok choy, mushrooms, ginger, garlic, and

chili. Simmer for 5 minutes, until bok choy is tender yet still crisp and mushrooms are softened. Add tomatoes, green onions, tofu, and carrot. Heat through for 1 minute. Stir in cilantro just before serving.

Baby Spinach Salad with Avocado, Olives, Feta, and Walnuts

Nutritional Information Per Serving
Net Carbs: 5.5 grams
Fiber: 7.5 grams
Protein: 8 grams
Fat: 28 grams
Calories: 315

Recipe Information
Makes: 1 serving
Prep Time: 0:08:00
Marinate Time: N/A
Cook Time: N/A
Cool Time: N/A

Ingredients
1 cup baby spinach
1 ounce feta cheese, drained and crumbled
7 walnut halves
½ avocado, diced
5 olives

Directions
Combine spinach with feta, avocado, and olives. Toss with low-carb dressing of your choice and season to taste with salt and freshly ground black pepper. Top with walnuts.

Alfredo Sauce

Nutritional Information Per Serving
Net Carbs: 2.0 grams
Fiber: 0.0 grams
Protein: 4.0 grams
Fat: 28.0 grams
Calories: 280

Recipe Information
Makes: 6 servings
Prep Time: N/A
Marinate Time: N/A
Cook Time: 0:10:00
Cool Time: 0:10:00

Ingredients
2 tablespoons unsalted butter
1½ cups heavy cream
½ cup grated Parmesan
¼ cup grated Pecorino Romano
1/8 teaspoon pepper
Pinch ground nutmeg

Directions

Melt butter in a medium saucepan over medium heat. Add cream and simmer until reduced to 1 cup, about 10 minutes. Remove from heat; stir in Parmesan, Pecorino Romano, pepper, and nutmeg until cheeses have melted and sauce is smooth. Serve right away over low-carb noodles or as a topping for chicken or steak.

Cauliflower Sour Cream Mash (Pseudo Mashed Potatoes)

Nutritional Information Per Serving
Net Carbs: 2.5 grams
Fiber: 2.5 grams
Protein: 3 grams
Fat: 6 grams
Calories: 77

Recipe Information
Makes: 6 servings
Prep Time: 0:10:00
Marinate Time: N/A
Cook Time: 0:10:00
Cool Time: N/A

Ingredients
1 cauliflower (2 pounds)
2 tablespoons sour cream
2 tablespoons heavy cream

1½ tablespoons butter

1 teaspoon salt

Directions

Add a cup of water to a large pot and insert a steamer basket. Place cauliflower florets in the basket and bring water to a boil over high heat. Cover tightly, cook until tender, 10–12 minutes, and drain. Purée cauliflower in a food processor, adding florets in batches. Add sour cream, heavy cream, butter, and salt; process until smooth and well combined. Reheat gently, if necessary, before serving.

Grilled Chicken and Vegetables with Fresh Basil

Nutritional Information Per Serving

Net Carbs: 8.5 grams

Fiber: 2 grams

Protein: 50.5 grams

Fat: 17 grams

Calories: 399

Recipe Information

Makes: 4 servings

Prep Time: 0:10:00

Marinate Time: 1:00:00

Cook Time: 0:15:00

Cool Time: N/A

Ingredients

¼ cup shallots, roughly chopped

3 tablespoons extra-virgin olive oil

1 tablespoon chopped garlic

1 teaspoon salt

½ teaspoon black pepper

2 pounds of skinless chicken breast halves

1 red bell pepper, seeded and quartered (about 1½ cups)

1 medium zucchini, quartered lengthwise (about 1½ cups)

1 medium yellow squash, quartered lengthwise (about 1½ cups)

1 medium leek, root trimmed, halved lengthwise

¼ cup fresh basil, chiffonade

Directions

Mix shallots, oil, garlic, salt, and pepper in a large, resealable plastic bag. Add chicken, peppers, zucchini, squash, and leek. Gently shake bag to coat chicken and vegetables, and marinate in refrigerator for 1 to 3 hours, turning occasionally. Prepare a medium-low grill. Place chicken on grill and cook until just cooked through, turning once, about 12 minutes. About 2 minutes into cooking process, add peppers and cook until tender, turning once, about 10 minutes. About 2 minutes after adding peppers, add zucchini, squash, and leeks and cook until tender, turning once, about 8 minutes. Sprinkle with basil before serving.

Grilled Steaks with Mustard-Herb Rub

Nutritional Information Per Serving
Net Carbs: 2 grams
Fiber: 0.5 grams
Protein: 46 grams
Fat: 19 grams
Calories: 377

Recipe Information
Makes: 4 servings
Prep Time: 0:10:00
Marinate Time: N/A
Cook Time: 0:10:00
Cool Time: N/A

Ingredients
2 tablespoons Dijon mustard
2 large garlic cloves, pushed through a press
½ teaspoon dried rosemary
½ teaspoon dried thyme
½ teaspoon dried oregano
½ teaspoon pepper
2 pounds of beef rib eye steaks or boneless top loin steaks, 1" thick

Directions
Combine mustard, garlic, rosemary, thyme, oregano, and pepper. Spread mixture on both sides of steaks. Grill steaks over medium coals or medium setting on gas grill, turning

occasionally, 11 to 14 minutes for medium-rare to medium (if using top loin steaks, grill a little longer), turning halfway through cooking time. Season with salt to taste.

Santa Fe Turkey Meatballs

Nutritional Information Per Serving
Net Carbs: 4 grams
Fiber: 2.5 grams
Protein: 32.5 grams
Fat: 26.5 grams
Calories: 390

Recipe Information
Makes: 4 servings
Prep Time: 0:20:00
Marinate Time: N/A
Cook Time: 0:20:00
Cool Time: N/A

Ingredients
1 tablespoon canola oil, divided
1 small onion, finely chopped (about ½ cup)
2 slices low-carb bread, torn into small pieces
¼ cup water
¼ cup heavy cream
1 pound ground turkey
1 teaspoon chopped garlic
1 teaspoon ground cumin

1 teaspoon salt

½ teaspoon freshly ground black pepper

¼ pound pepper Jack (or Monterey Jack) cheese, cut into 12 equal-sized cubes

½ cup chicken broth

½ cup prepared green salsa

Directions

In a large nonstick skillet, heat 1 teaspoon oil over medium heat. Sauté onion until softened, about 5 minutes, and set aside. In a large bowl, soak bread in water and cream until soft. Mix in turkey, garlic, cumin, salt, pepper, and onions. Divide mixture into 12 portions, insert a cheese cube into the center of each portion, and form into balls (make sure cheese is completely enclosed). Heat remaining oil over medium heat. Cook meatballs 5 minutes, turning to brown on all sides. Add salsa and chicken broth to skillet, reduce heat to medium-low, and simmer, covered until meatballs are cooked through, about 10 minutes. Transfer to a plate and spoon sauce over meatballs before serving.

Savory Key Lime Mousse

Nutritional Information Per Serving

Net Carbs: 4 grams

Fiber: 7 grams

Protein: 2 grams

Fat: 16 grams

Calories: 180

Recipe Information
Makes: 4 servings
Prep Time: 0:20:00
Marinate Time: N/A
Cook Time: 0:20:00
Cool Time: N/A

Ingredients
2 tablespoons extra-virgin olive oil
2 tablespoons fresh-squeezed lime juice
3 medium/large cloves garlic, pressed or minced
1 bunch asparagus (approximately 24 small or medium spears)
¼ teaspoon sea salt, or to taste
¼ teaspoon ground black pepper
½ teaspoon chili powder, preferably chipotle
¼ teaspoon ground cumin
½ cup diced red bell pepper
½ teaspoon lime zest,* loosely packed, optional
2 tablespoons finely chopped cilantro
1 teaspoon tamari, optional
2 tablespoons diced scallion, as garnish
2 teaspoons sesame seeds, preferably a combo of black and white, as garnish

Directions
Preheat the oven to 375°F. Place the olive oil, lime juice, and garlic in a 9-inch by 13-inch casserole dish and stir well. Cut off the tough bottom portion of the asparagus and put the spears in the casserole dish. Add the salt, ground pepper, chili powder, and cumin and toss well. Place the asparagus in the

oven and bake for 10 minutes. Remove from the oven and add the bell pepper and toss gently but well. Return to the oven and bake for an additional 10 minutes. Remove from the oven. Add the lime zest (if using), cilantro, and tamari (if using). Toss gently again. Garnish with green onion and sesame seeds before serving.

*To zest the lime, use a zester, microplane, or the fine portion of a box grater. Be careful to zest only the outer skin of the lime as the inner, white portion is bitter.

Keep in mind, again, that this is not an exhaustive list; experimentation is key, provided you stay within the allowable foods realm. Gloss over the above recipes and you will see *dozens* of ingredients strewn about that work in the Smoke Free Eating plan, so mix and match! You know you can eat any meat you want...season it any way you like with anything you see! Chicken? Marinate it in lemon juice, garlic, seasoning salt...slather it in butter and drop it on the barbecue for all I care! Playing around with the intention of discovering your favorites should be a fun exercise in culinary exploration, rather than a task, so enjoy it. Cooking can be wonderfully relaxing and there is always the added comfort of knowing that what's in your food is on the plan.

Appendix B:
Mini Carb Counter

Food Item

			Total Carbs (g)	Fiber (g)	Net Carbs (g)	Fat (g)	Pro-tein	Calo-ries
Fats, Oils & Dressings								
1.00	tsp	Corn Oil	0.0	0	0.0	4.5	0.0	40
1.00	tsp	Olive Oil	0.0	0	0.0	4.5	0.0	40
1.00	tsp	Sesame Oil	0.0	0	0.0	4.5	0.0	40
1.00	tsp	Mayonnaise	0.1	0	0.1	3.7	0.1	33
2.00	tbs	Salad Dressing, Blue Cheese	2.3	0	2.3	16.0	1.5	154
2.00	tbs	Salad Dressing, Caesar	0.6	0.1	0.5	10.5	2.8	107
2.00	tbs	Salad Dressing, Italian	3.0	0	3.0	14.2	0.2	137
2.00	tbs	Salad Dressing, Ranch	1.4	0	1.4	11.3	0.9	109
2.00	tbs	Salad Dressing, Thousand Island	4.8	0	4.8	11.2	0.3	118

Gravies & Sauces

			Total Carbs (g)	Fiber (g)	Net Carbs (g)	Fat (g)	Protein	Calories
2.00	tbs	Barbecue Sauce	4.0	0.4	3.6	0.6	0.6	23
1.00	tbs	Easy Barbecue Sauce*	1.6	0.0	1.6			
0.25	cup	Gravy, au jus	1.5	0.0	1.5	0.1	0.7	10
0.25	cup	Gravy, canned (chicken, beef, etc)	3.2	0.2	3.0	3.4	1.1	47
2.00	tbs	Hollandaise Sauce	0.3	0.0	0.3	9.1	1.0	85
1.00	tbs	Ketchup Cookup*	1.0	0.25	0.75			
0.25	cup	Spaghetti/ Marinara Sauce	5.1	1.0	4.1	1.3	0.9	36
0.25	cup	Sweet & Sour Sauce	15.1	0.1	15.1	0.0	0.2	59
2.00	tbs	Tartar Sauce	1.2	0.1	1.1	16.4	0.4	149
2.00	tbs	Teriyaki Sauce	5.7	0.0	5.7	0.0	2.1	30
0.25	cup	Tomato Sauce	4.4	0.9	3.5	0.1	0.8	18

Food Item

Condiments

			Total Carbs (g)	Fiber (g)	Net Carbs (g)	Fat (g)	Protein	Calories
1.00	tbs	Balsamic Vinegar	2.3	0.0	2.3	0.0	0.1	10
1.00	tbs	Capers	0.4	0.3	0.1	0.1	0.2	2
1.00	tsp	Chili Powder	1.4	0.9	0.5	0.4	0.3	8
1.00	tbs	Cider Vinegar	0.9	0.0	0.9	0.0	0.0	2
2.00	tbs	Cranberry Sauce	13.5	0.3	13.1	0.1	0.1	52

1.00	tsp	Cumin	0.8	0.7	0.1	0.5	0.4	9
1.00	tsp	Dijon Mustard	0.6	0.1	0.5	0.5	0.3	6
1.00	each	Dill Pickle	2.7	0.8	1.9	0.1	0.4	12
1.00	tsp	Fish Sauce	0.2	0.0	0.2	0.0	0.3	2
1.00	each	Garlic	1.0	0.1	0.9	0.0	0.2	4
1.00	tbs	Ginger, Root Slices	0.9	0.1	0.8	0.0	0.1	4
1.00	tsp	Honey	5.8	0.0	5.8	0.0	0.0	21
1.00	tsp	Horseradish-Prepared	0.6	0.2	0.4	0.0	0.1	2
1.00	tsp	Jam	4.6	0.1	4.5	0.0	0.0	19
1.00	tsp	Jelly	4.5	0.1	4.4	0.0	0.0	18
1.00	tbs	Ketchup/Catsup	4.2	0.2	4.0	0.1	0.2	16
1.00	tbs	Maple Syrup	13.4	0.0	13.4	0.0	0.0	52
2.00	tbs	Mint Sauce*	2.3	0.3	2.0			
1.00	tbs	Miso Paste	3.0	0.4	2.6	0.8	1.9	27
5.00	each	Olives, black	1.4	0.7	0.7	2.3	0.2	25
5.00	each	Olives, green	2.5	0.0	2.5	5.0	0.0	50
1.00	tbs	Pesto Sauce	1.0	0.4	0.6	7.1	2.8	78
1.00	tbs	Pickle Relish	5.4	0.2	5.2	0.1	0.1	20
1.00	tsp	Preserves	4.6	0.1	4.5	0.0	0.0	19
1.00	tbs	Red Wine Vinegar	0.0	0.0	0.0	0.0	0.0	0
1.00	tbs	Rice Vinegar, seasoned	3.0	0.0	3.0	0.0	0.0	12
1.00	tbs	Salsa, green	0.6	0.1	0.6	0.0	0.2	4
1.00	tbs	Salsa, red	0.8	0.1	0.7	0.0	0.1	4
1.00	tbs	Sherry vinegar	0.9	0.0	0.9	0.0	0.0	2
1.00	tbs	Soy sauce	1.0	0.1	0.9	0.0	1.9	11

1.00	tbs	Soy Sauce-Low	1.4	0.1	1.2	0.0	0.8	8
1.00	tbs	Tahini	3.2	0.7	2.5	8.0	2.6	89
1.00	tbs	White Wine Vinegar	1.5	0.0	1.5	0.0	0.0	5
1.00	tsp	Worcestershire Sauce	0.9	0.0	0.9	0.0	0.0	4

Food Item

			Total Carbs (g)	Fiber (g)	Net Carbs (g)	Fat (g)	Pro-tein	Calo-ries

Dairy – Cheese, Butter, Cream, Milk & Yogurt

1.00	piece	American Cheese, 2/3 oz. slice	0.3	0	0.3	6.6	4.7	79
2.00	tbs	Blue Cheese, crumbled	0.4	0	0.4	4.8	3.6	60
2.00	tbs	Cheddar Cheese-Shredded	0.2	0	0.2	4.7	3.5	57
2.00	tbs	Cream Cheese	0.8	0	0.8	10.1	2.2	101
0.50	cup	Creamed Cottage Cheese Small Curd	2.8	0	2.8	4.7	13.1	109
2.00	tbs	Feta Cheese, crumbled	0.8	0	0.8	4.0	2.7	49
2.00	tbs	Fontina Cheese-Shredded	0.2	0	0.2	4.2	3.5	53
2.00	tbs	Goat Cheese-Soft Type	0.3	0	0.3	6.5	5.7	82

1.00	oz-wt	Mascarpone	0.6	0	0.6	13.2	2.0	126
2.00	tbs	Monterey Jack Cheese Shredded	0.1	0	0.1	4.3	3.5	53
2.00	tbs	Mozzarella Cheese-Whole Milk	0.3	0	0.3	3.1	2.7	40
2.00	tbs	Parmesan Cheese-Shredded	0.3	0	0.3	2.7	3.8	42
1.00	oz-wt	Provolone Cheese-Diced	0.6	0	0.6	7.5	7.3	100
0.25	cup	Ricotta Cheese-Whole Milk	1.9	0	1.9	8.0	6.9	107
2.00	tbs	Swiss Cheese-Shredded	0.5	0	0.5	3.7	3.8	51
1.00	tsp	Butter	0.0	0	0.0	3.8	0.0	34
1.00	tsp	Whipped Butter	0.0	0	0.0	2.6	0.0	23
1.00	cup	Buttermilk, 1% low fat	13.0	0	13.0	2.5	9.0	110
2.00	tbs	Half and Half Cream	1.0	0	1.0	3.0	1.0	40
2.00	tbs	Heavy Whipping Cream	0.8	0	0.8	11.0	0.6	103
2.00	tbs	Sour Cream	1.2	0	1.2	6.0	0.9	62
1.00	cup	Milk, 2%	11.7	0	11.7	4.7	8.1	121
1.00	cup	Milk, Whole	11.4	0	11.4	8.1	8.0	150
1.00	cup	Yogurt, low fat, plain	17.2	0	17.2	3.8	12.9	155
1.00	cup	Yogurt, whole milk, plain	11.4	0	11.4	8.0	8.5	150

Food Item

			Total Carbs (g)	Fiber (g)	Net Carbs (g)	Fat (g)	Pro-tein	Calo-ries

Beef & Veal

			Total Carbs (g)	Fiber (g)	Net Carbs (g)	Fat (g)	Pro-tein	Calo-ries
6.00	oz-wt	Beef Brisket	0.0	0	0.0	43.2	41.8	569
6.00	oz-wt	Beef Chuck	0.0	0	0.0	31.6	50.1	498
6.00	oz-wt	Beef Eye Round	0.0	0	0.0	24.0	45.2	410
6.00	oz-wt	Beef Short Ribs	0.0	0	0.0	71.4	36.7	801
6.00	oz-wt	Beef Tenderloin	0.0	0	0.0	41.8	40.7	551
6.00	oz-wt	Beef, Ground, Chuck	0.0	0	0.0	44.0	38.9	562
6.00	oz-wt	Beef, Ground, Round	0.0	0	0.0	28.1	46.7	454
6.00	oz-wt	Calf Liver	10.4	0	10.4	9.9	40.5	304
6.00	oz-wt	Chuck Eye Steak	0.0	0	0.0	41.1	46.2	568
6.00	oz-wt	Corned Beef Brisket	0.3	0	0.3	33.8	33.3	449
2.00	oz-wt	Frankfurter, Beef	1.1	0	1.1	16.6	7.2	185
6.00	oz-wt	Raw Boneless: Beef Steak -Shell- All-Lean-1/4"Trim-Brld	0.0	0	0.0	11.8	36.0	261
6.00	oz-wt	Prime Rib	0.0	0	0.0	56.4	36.9	667
6.00	oz-wt	Rib Eye Roast	0.0	0	0.0	37.8	42.4	522
6.00	oz-wt	Rib Eye Steak	0.0	0	0.0	19.9	47.7	383
6.00	oz-wt	Roast Beef, Deli	2.3	0	2.3	5.2	34.3	193

		Food Item	Total Carbs (g)	Fiber (g)	Net Carbs (g)	Fat (g)	Pro-tein	Calo-ries
6.00	oz-wt	Sirloin Steak	0.0	0	0.0	13.6	51.7	344
6.00	oz-wt	Skirt Steak	0.0	0	0.0	54.7	61.6	758
6.00	oz-wt	Top Loin	0.0	0	0.0	12.1	51.0	327
6.00	oz-wt	Top Sirloin	0.0	0	0.0	30.4	44.2	463
6.00	oz-wt	Veal Arm Shoulder	0.0	0	0.0	13.1	40.4	291
6.00	oz-wt	Veal Breast	0.0	0	0.0	33.5	39.6	472
6.00	oz-wt	Veal Cutlet	0.0	0	0.0	30.4	53.4	502
6.00	oz-wt	Veal, ground	0.0	0	0.0	12.9	41.5	293
6.00	oz-wt	Veal Loin	0.0	0	0.0	30.4	53.4	502
6.00	oz-wt	Veal Rib Chop	0.0	0	0.0	22.2	38.0	362
6.00	oz-wt	Veal Round Steak	0.0	0	0.0	7.0	47.6	265
6.00	oz-wt	Veal Scallops	0.0	0	0.0	6.3	52.2	279
6.00	oz-wt	Veal Shank	0.0	0	0.0	7.9	43.4	256
6.00	oz-wt	Veal Stew Meat	0.0	0	0.0	13.4	40.2	292

Food Item

			Total Carbs (g)	Fiber (g)	Net Carbs (g)	Fat (g)	Pro-tein	Calo-ries

Lamb

			Total Carbs (g)	Fiber (g)	Net Carbs (g)	Fat (g)	Pro-tein	Calo-ries
6.00	oz-wt	Lamb, ground	0.0	0	0.0	30.3	38.2	436
6.00	oz-wt	Lamb Rib Chops	0.0	0	0.0	50.3	37.6	614
6.00	oz-wt	Lamb Shoulder	0.0	0	0.0	12.6	46.2	312
6.00	oz-wt	Lamb Stew Meat	0.0	0	0.0	15.0	57.3	379
6.00	oz-wt	Leg of Lamb, bone in	0.0	0	0.0	8.2	30.0	203
6.00	oz-wt	Rack of Lamb, bone in	0.0	0	0.0	9.9	19.5	173

Pork

3.00	piece	Bacon	0.1	0	0.1	9.4	5.8	109
3.00	piece	Canadian Bacon	0.9	0	0.9	5.9	16.9	129
6.00	oz-wt	Ground Pork	0.0	0	0.0	33.4	41.4	478
6.00	oz-wt	Ham, boneless	0.0	0	0.0	15.3	38.5	303
2.00	oz-wt	Kielbasa	0.8	0	0.8	17.2	7.6	191
1.00	oz-wt	Pancetta	0.2	0	0.2	14.0	8.6	163
6.00	oz-wt	Pork Chop, center cut	0.0	0	0.0	9.7	34.9	237
2.00	oz-wt	Pork frankfurter	1.4	0	1.4	16.5	6.4	181
6.00	oz-wt	Pork Loin Chops	0.0	0	0.0	32.4	27.9	412
6.00	oz-wt	Pork Loin Roast	0.0	0	0.0	19.7	36.4	333
6.00	oz-wt	Pork loin, boneless	0.0	0	0.0	24.9	46.1	422
2.00	each	Pork Sausage	2.0	0	2.0	34.4	26.8	433
6.00	oz-wt	Pork Spareribs	0.0	0	0.0	51.5	49.4	675
6.00	oz-wt	Pork Tenderloin	0.0	0	0.0	8.2	47.9	279
6.00	oz-wt	Prosciutto	0.9	0	0.9	13.0	37.4	281

Lunch Meats

3.00	oz-wt	Beef Bologna	0.7	0	0.7	24.2	10.4	265
3.00	oz-wt	Beef Salami	2.4	0	2.4	17.6	12.8	223
3.00	oz-wt	Beef Pastrami	2.6	0	2.6	24.8	14.7	297

			Total Carbs (g)	Fiber (g)	Net Carbs (g)	Fat (g)	Pro-tein	Calo-ries
3.00	oz-wt	Pork Bologna	0.6	0	0.6	16.9	13.0	210
3.00	oz-wt	Pork Salami	1.4	0	1.4	28.7	19.2	346
3.00	oz-wt	Turkey Bologna	0.8	0	0.8	12.9	11.7	169
3.00	oz-wt	Turkey Breast	0.0	0	0.0	6.0	21.3	162
3.00	oz-wt	Turkey Roll	0.5	0	0.5	6.1	15.9	125

Food Item

			Total Carbs (g)	Fiber (g)	Net Carbs (g)	Fat (g)	Pro-tein	Calo-ries

Seafood

			Total Carbs (g)	Fiber (g)	Net Carbs (g)	Fat (g)	Pro-tein	Calo-ries
1.00	oz-wt	Anchovies in Oil-Drained	0.0	0	0.0	2.8	8.2	60
6.00	oz-wt	Bluefish	0.0	0	0.0	9.3	43.7	270
6.00	oz-wt	Catfish	0.0	0	0.0	17.2	35.3	306
6.00	oz-wt	Clams, canned	8.7	0	8.7	3.3	43.5	252
6.00	oz-wt	Cod	0.0	0	0.0	1.5	38.8	179
3.00	oz-wt	Cod, salted	0.0	0	0.0	2.0	53.4	247
6.00	oz-wt	Conch	26.4	0	26.4	1.4	81.1	468
6.00	oz-wt	Crab meat	0.0	0	0.0	3.0	34.4	174
6.00	oz-wt	Crab, canned	0.0	0	0.0	2.1	34.9	168
6.00	oz-wt	Crab, steamed	0.0	0	0.0	3.0	34.4	174
6.00	oz-wt	Halibut	0.0	0	0.0	5.2	47.2	249
6.00	oz-wt	Lobster meat	2.2	0	2.2	1.0	34.9	167
6.00	oz-wt	Lobster, whole	2.2	0	2.2	1.0	34.9	167
6.00	oz-wt	Mackerel	0.0	0	0.0	30.3	40.6	446
6.00	oz-wt	MahiMahi	0.0	0	0.0	1.6	42.0	193

			Total Carbs (g)	Fiber (g)	Net Carbs (g)	Fat (g)	Pro-tein	Calo-ries
6.00	oz-wt	Oysters	12.5	0	12.5	3.5	11.8	134
6.00	oz-wt	Salmon steak	0.0	0	0.0	24.6	45.1	415
6.00	oz-wt	Salmon, smoked	0.0	0	0.0	7.3	31.1	199
6.00	oz-wt	Scallops	3.9	0	3.9	5.4	27.7	182
6.00	oz-wt	Scrod	0.0	0	0.0	1.5	38.8	179
6.00	oz-wt	Shrimp	0.0	0	0.0	1.8	35.6	168
6.00	oz-wt	Smoked fish	0.0	0	0.0	34.3	30.0	437
6.00	oz-wt	Snapper	0.0	0	0.0	3.0	46.5	227
6.00	oz-wt	Squid	7.0	0	7.0	3.1	35.3	209
6.00	oz-wt	Trout	0.0	0	0.0	12.2	41.3	287
6.00	oz-wt	Tuna filet	0.0	0	0.0	2.2	53.0	245
6.00	oz-wt	Tuna steak	0.0	0	0.0	2.2	53.0	245
6.00	oz-wt	Tuna, canned, oil packed	0.0	0	0.0	14.0	49.6	337
6.00	oz-wt	Tuna, canned, wa-ter packed	0.0	0	0.0	1.4	43.4	197

Food Item

			Total Carbs (g)	Fiber (g)	Net Carbs (g)	Fat (g)	Pro-tein	Calo-ries

Poultry & Eggs

6.00	oz-wt	Chicken Breast Cutlet	0.0	0	0.0	12.7	48.7	322
6.00	oz-wt	Chicken Breast, boneless	0.0	0	0.0	12.7	48.7	322
1.00	each	Chicken Leg	0.0	0	0.0	15.4	29.7	265
1.00	each	Chicken Thigh	0.0	0	0.0	9.6	15.5	153

6.00	oz-wt	Chicken Thigh,	0.0	0	0.0	34.6	39.2	479
6.00	oz-wt	Chicken thigh, skinless, boneless	0.0	0	0.0	8.9	44.6	270
1.00	each	Chicken Wing	0.0	0	0.0	6.6	9.1	99
6.00	oz-wt	Chicken, ground	0.0	0	0.0	22.5	40.2	374
6.00	oz-wt	Chicken, light and dark, roasted	0.0	0	0.0	12.6	49.2	323
6.00	oz-wt	Chicken, whole	0.1	0	0.1	14.7	29.8	260
2.00	oz-wt	Chicken/turkey sausage	0.3	0	0.3	6.4	9.6	97
6.00	oz-wt	Cornish Game Hen	0.0	0	0.0	26.1	31.9	372
6.00	oz-wt	Duck breast, skinless	0.0	0	0.0	9.6	45.0	279
6.00	oz-wt	Duck, whole	0.0	0	0.0	89.2	26.1	916
6.00	oz-wt	Goose, whole	0.0	0	0.0	23.6	27.1	329
6.00	oz-wt	Turkey breast cutlet	0.0	0	0.0	1.5	59.3	266
6.00	oz-wt	Turkey Breast, skinless, boneless	0.0	0	0.0	1.5	59.3	266
6.00	oz-wt	Turkey, ground	0.0	0	0.0	21.2	44.1	378
6.00	oz-wt	Turkey, whole	0.1	0	0.1	12.2	36.1	264
1.00	each	Egg white	0.3	0	0.3	0.0	3.5	17
1.00	each	Egg Yolk	0.3	0	0.3	5.1	2.8	59
1.00	each	Egg whole	0.6	0	0.6	5.3	6.3	78

Food Item

			Total Carbs (g)	Fiber (g)	Net Carbs (g)	Fat (g)	Pro-tein	Calo-ries
Tofu, Beans and Grains								
8.00	fl oz	Soy Milk	4.4	3.2	1.2	4.7	6.7	81
4.00	oz-wt	Tofu, firm	4.9	2.6	2.2	9.9	17.9	164
4.00	oz-wt	Tofu, silken	3.3	0.1	3.2	3.1	5.4	62
0.50	cup	Baby Lima Beans	21.2	7.0	14.2	0.3	7.3	115
0.50	cup	Black Beans	20.4	7.5	12.9	0.5	7.6	114
0.50	cup	Blackeyed Peas	17.9	5.6	12.3	0.5	6.6	100
0.50	cup	CA Red Kidney Beans	19.8	8.2	11.6	0.1	8.1	110
0.50	cup	Chickpea/ Garbanzo Beans	22.5	6.2	16.2	2.1	7.3	134
0.50	cup	Great Northern Beans	18.7	6.2	12.5	0.4	7.4	104
2.00	tbs	Hummos/Hummus	6.2	1.6	4.6	2.6	1.5	53
0.50	cup	Lentils	19.9	7.8	12.1	0.4	8.9	115
0.50	cup	Navy Beans	23.9	5.8	18.1	0.5	7.9	129
0.50	cup	Pink Beans	23.6	4.5	19.1	0.4	7.7	126
0.50	cup	Pinto Beans	18.0	7.0	11.0	1.0	7.0	110
0.50	cup	Soybeans	9.9	3.8	6.2	5.8	11.1	127
0.50	cup	Bulgur Wheat-Cooked	16.9	4.1	12.8	0.2	2.8	76
2.00	tbs	Cornmeal	11.7	1.1	10.6	0.5	1.2	55
0.50	cup	Couscous-Cooked	18.2	1.1	17.1	0.1	3.0	88
0.50	cup	Hominy-Cooked	11.8	2.1	9.7	0.7	1.2	59
0.50	cup	Kasha-Cooked	74.3	9.4	64.8	2.7	11.6	343

			Total Carbs (g)	Fiber (g)	Net Carbs (g)	Fat (g)	Protein	Calories
2.00	tbs	Oat Bran-Dry	7.8	1.8	6.0	0.8	2.0	29
0.50	cup	Pearled Barley-Cooked	22.2	3.0	19.2	0.3	1.8	97
0.25	cup	Quinoa Grain-Dry	29.3	2.5	26.8	2.5	5.6	159
0.50	cup	Rice, brown, cooked	22.4	1.8	20.6	0.9	2.5	108
0.50	cup	Rice, white, cooked	22.3	0.3	21.9	0.2	2.1	103
0.50	cup	Rice, wild, cooked	17.5	1.5	16.0	0.3	3.3	83
2.00	tbs	Wheat Germ-Toasted	7.0	1.8	5.2	1.5	4.1	54

Food Item

			Total Carbs (g)	Fiber (g)	Net Carbs (g)	Fat (g)	Protein	Calories

Nuts & Seeds

			Total Carbs (g)	Fiber (g)	Net Carbs (g)	Fat (g)	Protein	Calories
2.00	tbs	Almond Butter	6.8	1.2	5.6	18.9	4.8	203
2.00	tbs	Almonds, slivered	3.3	1.6	1.7	8.6	3.5	102
2.00	tbs	Almonds, whole	3.6	2.2	1.4	8.9	3.7	106
6.00	each	Chestnuts, roasted	26.7	2.6	24.2	1.1	1.6	124
2.00	tbs	Hazelnuts, Chopped	2.4	1.4	1.0	8.7	2.1	90
2.00	tbs	Hazelnuts, Whole	2.8	1.6	1.2	10.3	2.5	106
2.00	tbs	Macadamia Nuts	2.3	1.4	0.9	12.7	1.3	120
2.00	tbs	Peanut Butter, natural	6.9	2.1	4.8	15.9	7.7	187

2.00	tbs	Peanut Butter,	6.2	1.9	4.3	16.3	8.1	190
2.00	tbs	Peanuts	3.4	1.7	1.8	8.9	4.7	105
2.00	tbs	Pecans, chopped	2.1	1.4	0.6	10.7	1.4	103
2.00	tbs	Pine Nuts	2.4	0.8	1.7	8.6	4.1	96
2.00	tbs	Pistachio Nuts	4.7	1.6	3.1	6.9	3.3	88
2.00	tbs	Pumpkin Seeds	3.1	0.7	2.4	7.9	4.2	93
2.00	tbs	Sunflower Seeds	3.4	1.9	1.5	8.9	4.1	103
2.00	tbs	Walnuts, chopped	2.1	1.0	1.1	9.8	2.3	98
2.00	tbs	Walnuts, halves	1.7	0.8	0.9	8.2	1.9	82
0.50	cup	Couscous-Cooked	18.2	1.1	17.1	0.1	3.0	88
0.50	cup	Hominy-Cooked	11.8	2.1	9.7	0.7	1.2	59
0.50	cup	Kasha-Cooked	74.3	9.4	64.8	2.7	11.6	343
0.50	cup	Millet-Cooked	28.4	1.6	26.8	1.2	4.2	143
2.00	tbs	Oat Bran-Dry	7.8	1.8	6.0	0.8	2.0	29
0.50	cup	Pearled Barley-Cooked	22.2	3.0	19.2	0.3	1.8	97
0.25	cup	Quinoa Grain-Dry	29.3	2.5	26.8	2.5	5.6	159
0.50	cup	Rice, brown, cooked	22.4	1.8	20.6	0.9	2.5	108
0.50	cup	Rice, white, cooked	22.3	0.3	21.9	0.2	2.1	103
0.50	cup	Rice, wild, cooked	17.5	1.5	16.0	0.3	3.3	83
2.00	tbs	Wheat Germ-Toasted	7.0	1.8	5.2	1.5	4.1	54

Food Item

			Total Carbs (g)	Fiber (g)	Net Carbs (g)	Fat (g)	Pro-tein	Calo-ries

Cereals

			Total Carbs (g)	Fiber (g)	Net Carbs (g)	Fat (g)	Pro-tein	Calo-ries
1.00	cup	Corn Flakes	24.2	0.8	23.4	0.2	1.8	102
0.50	cup	Cream of Rice Cereal-Cooked	13.9	0.1	13.8	0.1	1.1	63
0.50	cup	Cream of Wheat -Cooked	15.8	1.4	14.3	0.2	2.2	77
0.50	cup	Oatmeal-Cooked	12.6	2.0	10.6	1.2	3.0	73
1.00	cup	Puffed Wheat Cereal	11.1	0.6	10.5	0.2	2.1	51
1.00	cup	Raisin Bran	47.1	8.2	38.9	1.5	5.6	186
1.00	cup	Rice Krispies	22.8	0.3	22.5	0.3	1.7	100

Soups

			Total Carbs (g)	Fiber (g)	Net Carbs (g)	Fat (g)	Pro-tein	Calo-ries
1.00	cup	Broth, beef	1.0	0.0	1.0	1.4	4.8	38
1.00	cup	Broth, chicken	1.5	0.0	1.5	1.5	3.1	31
1.00	cup	Soup, black bean	19.8	4.4	15.4	1.5	5.6	116
1.00	cup	Soup, chicken noodle	9.4	0.7	8.6	2.5	4.0	75
1.00	cup	Soup, cream of potato	17.2	0.5	16.7	6.4	5.8	149
1.00	cup	Soup, cream of tomato	22.3	2.7	19.6	6.0	6.1	161
1.00	cup	Soup, minestrone	11.2	1.0	10.3	2.5	4.3	82

1.00	cup	Soup, New England	16.6	1.5	15.1	6.6	9.5	164
1.00	cup	Soup, onion	8.2	1.0	7.2	1.7	3.8	58
1.00	cup	Soup, vegetable	19.0	1.2	17.8	3.7	3.5	122

Pasta

0.50	cup	Noodles, egg, cooked	19.9	0.9	19.0	1.2	3.8	106
0.50	cup	Pasta, spinach, cooked	18.3	2.5	15.9	0.4	3.2	91
0.50	cup	Pasta, whole wheat, cooked	18.6	2.0	16.6	0.4	3.7	87
0.50	cup	Pasta/Noodles, dry, cooked	19.8	1.2	18.6	0.5	3.3	99
4.00	oz-wt	Pasta/Noodles, fresh, cooked	28.3	2.0	26.3	1.2	5.8	149

Snacks

10.00	piece	Potato Chips	10.6	0.9	9.7	6.9	1.4	107
10.00	piece	Pretzels	47.5	1.9	45.6	2.1	5.5	229
0.50	oz-wt	Soy Nuts	4.5	2.5	2.0	2.0	6.0	60
10.00	piece	Tortilla Chips	11.3	1.2	10.2	4.7	1.3	90

Food Item

			Total Carbs (g)	Fiber (g)	Net Carbs (g)	Fat (g)	Pro- tein	Calo- ries
Breads, Rolls & Crackers								
1.00	each	Bagel, 2 1/2 oz	38.0	1.7	36.3	1.1	7.5	195
1.00	each	Biscuit, 2 oz	27.6	1.0	26.6	6.9	4.2	191
1.00	each	Blueberry Muffin, 2 oz	27.4	1.5	25.9	3.7	3.1	158
1.00	each	Bran Muffin, 2 oz	23.8	4.0	19.8	7.3	4.0	164
1.00	each	Breadsticks, sesa- me, small	2.2	0.1	2.1	0.5	0.4	15
1.00	each	Corn Muffin, 2 oz	29.0	1.9	27.1	4.8	3.4	174
1.00	piece	Cornbread 2.5 x 2.5 x 1.5 pce	22.7	1.9	20.7	4.9	4.0	152
5.00	each	Crackers, butter-type	51.4	1.5	49.8	18.3	5.83	93
5.00	each	Crackers, rye wafers	44.2	12.6	31.6	0.5	5.3	184
5.00	each	Crackers, saltines	10.7	0.5	10.3	1.8	1.4	65
5.00	each	Crackers, water	10.0	0.6	9.4	0.0	1.3	44
1.00	each	Croissant	27.0	0.0	27.0	17.0	4.0	270
1.00	each	English Muffin	26.0	1.5	24.5	1.0	4.4	133
1.00	each	Hard White Roll	30.0	1.3	28.7	2.5	5.6	167
1.00	piece	Italian Bread	15.0	0.8	14.2	1.1	2.6	81
1.00	each	Pita Pocket Bread, 6 1/2"diameter	33.4	1.3	32.1	0.7	5.5	165
1.00	each	Popover	10.4	0.3	10.1	1.5	2.6	67

1.00	piece	Pumpernickel	12.4	1.7	10.7	0.8	2.3	65
1.00	piece	Raisin Bread	13.6	1.1	12.5	1.1	2.1	71
1.00	piece	Rye Bread	15.5	1.9	13.6	1.1	2.7	83
1.00	each	Soft Hoagie Roll	32.0	2.0	30.0	4.5	7.0	200
1.00	piece	Sourdough Bread	13.0	0.8	12.2	0.8	2.2	69
1.00	each	Tortilla, corn	12.1	1.4	10.8	0.7	1.5	58
1.00	each	Tortillas, flour, 8"	25.3	0.0	25.3	3.1	4.4	146
1.00	piece	Wheat Bread	11.8	1.1	10.7	1.0	2.3	65
1.00	piece	White Bread	14.9	0.7	14.2	1.1	2.5	80
1.00	piec	Whole grain bread	11.8	1.1	10.7	1.0	2.3	65

Food Item

			Total Carbs (g)	Fiber (g)	Net Carbs (g)	Fat (g)	Pro-tein	Calo-ries

Baking Products

2.00	tbs	All Purpose White Flour	11.9	0.4	11.5	0.2	1.6	57
1.00	oz-wt	Baking Chocolate, unsweetened	8.0	4.4	3.7	15.7	2.9	148
0.50	tsp	Baking Powder	0.6	0.0	0.6	0.0	0.0	1
0.50	tsp	Baking Soda	0.0	0.0	0.0	0.0	0.0	0
2.00	tbs	Chocolate Chips, semisweet	13.3	1.2	12.0	6.3	0.9	101
0.50	tsp	Cinnamon	0.9	0.6	0.3	0.0	0.0	3
0.50	tsp	Cocoa Powder, unsweetened	0.5	0.3	0.2	0.1	0.2	3

2.00	tbs	Coconut	0.8	0.3	0.5	6.0	0.6	56
2.00	tbs	Coconut, dried, unsweetened	2.4	1.6	0.8	6.3	0.7	64
2.00	tbs	Cornmeal	13.4	1.3	12.1	0.3	1.5	63
1.00	each	Gelatin, unsweetened	0.0	0.0	0.0	0.0	6.0	23
1.00	tsp	Ghee	0.0	0.0	0.0	4.2	0.0	37
1.00	tsp	Margarine	0.0	0.0	0.0	3.8	0.0	34
1.00	tbs	Molasses	12.5	0.0	12.5	0.0	0.0	48
1.00	tsp	Sugar, brown	4.5	0.0	4.5	0.0	0.0	17
1.00	tsp	Sugar, white	4.2	0.0	4.2	0.0	0.0	16
1.00	each	Popover	10.4	0.3	10.1	1.5	2.6	67
1.00	piece	Pumpernickel Bread	12.4	1.7	10.7	0.8	2.3	65
1.00	piece	Raisin Bread	13.6	1.1	12.5	1.1	2.1	71
1.00	piece	Rye Bread	15.5	1.9	13.6	1.1	2.7	83
1.00	each	Soft Hoagie Roll	32.0	2.0	30.0	4.5	7.0	200
1.00	piece	Sourdough Bread	13.0	0.8	12.2	0.8	2.2	69
1.00	each	Tortilla, corn	12.1	1.4	10.8	0.7	1.5	58
1.00	each	Tortillas, flour, 8"	25.3	0.0	25.3	3.1	4.4	146
1.00	piece	Wheat Bread	11.8	1.1	10.7	1.0	2.3	65
1.00	piece	White Bread	14.9	0.7	14.2	1.1	2.5	80
1.00	piec	Whole grain bread	11.8	1.1	10.7	1.0	2.3	65

Pancakes, Waffles & French Toast

1.00	piece	French Toast-Frozen	18.9	0.7	18.3	3.6	4.4	126
1.00	each	Pancakes-Frozen-Ready To Eat 6"	31.8	1.3	30.5	2.4	3.8	167

1.00	each	Pancakes-	21.8	1.1	20.7	7.5	4.9	175
1.00	each	Waffles-Frozen-4" square	13.5	0.8	12.7	2.7	2.1	88
1.00	each	Waffles-Home-made-7" diam	24.7	1.1	23.6	10.6	5.9	218

Desserts & Pastries

1.00	piece	Cake, angelfood, 1/12 cake	29.4	0.1	29.2	0.2	3.1	129
1.00	piece	Cake, chocolate layer, 3 oz slice	38.0	2.0	36.0	16.0	2.0	300
1.00	piece	Cake, coffeecake, 2 oz slice	29.6	0.7	28.9	5.4	3.1	178
1.00	piece	Cake, pound cake, 1 oz slice	13.8	0.1	13.7	5.6	1.6	110
1.00	oz-wt	Chocolate, dark	17.9	1.7	16.2	8.5	1.2	136
1.00	oz-wt	Chocolate, milk	16.8	1.0	15.8	8.7	2.0	145
1.00	each	Cookie, chocolate chip, 1/2 oz	10.3	0.2	10.0	4.1	0.9	79
1.00	each	Cookie, oatmeal, 1/2 oz	12.4	0.5	11.9	3.3	1.1	81
1.00	each	Cookie, peanut butter, 2/3 oz	11.8	0.4	11.4	4.8	1.8	95
1.00	each	Cookie, sugar, 1/2 oz	10.2	0.1	10.1	3.2	0.8	72
1.00	each	Doughnut, glazed	26.6	0.7	25.9	13.7	3.8	242
1.00	each	Doughnut, plain	19.0	1.0	18.0	11.0	3.0	180
0.50	cup	Ice cream, chocolate	18.6	0.8	17.8	7.3	2.5	143
0.50	cup	Ice cream, fruit	18.2	0.2	18.0	5.5	2.1	127

1.00	piece	Pie, apple, 1/8 of 9" pie	57.5	2.2	55.3	19.4	3.7	411
1.00	piece	Pie, cherry, 1/8 of 9" pie	69.3	2.7	66.6	22.0	5.0	486
1.00	piece	Pie, lemon meringue, 1/6 8" pie	53.3	1.4	52.0	9.8	1.7	303
1.00	piece	Pie, pecan, 1/8 of 9" pie	63.7	6.1	57.6	27.1	6.0	503
1.00	piece	Pie, pumpkin, 1/8 of 9" pie	40.9	4.2	36.7	14.4	7.0	316

Food Item

			Total Carbs (g)	Fiber (g)	Net Carbs (g)	Fat (g)	Pro-tein	Calo-ries

Herbs

1.00	tbs	Basil, fresh	0.1	0.1	0.0	0.0	0.1	1
1.00	tbs	Chives, fresh	0.1	0.1	0.1	0.0	0.1	1
1.00	tbs	Cilantro (Chinese Parsley)	0.1	0.1	0.0	0.0	0.1	1
1.00	tbs	Dill, fresh	0.0	0.0	0.0	0.0	0.0	0
1.00	tbs	Parsley, fresh	0.2	0.1	0.1	0.0	0.1	1

Food Item

Fruit & Fruit Juices

			Total Carbs (g)	Fiber (g)	Net Carbs (g)	Fat (g)	Pro-tein	Calo-ries
1.00	each	Apple, medium	21.0	3.7	17.3	0.5	0.3	81
0.25	cup	Applesauce	6.9	0.7	6.2	0.0	0.1	26
0.25	cup	Apricots, dried	24.9	3.6	21.3	0.2	1.5	96
1.00	each	Apricots, fresh	3.9	0.8	3.1	0.1	0.5	17
1.00	each	Avocado	14.9	10.1	4.8	30.8	4.0	324
1.00	each	Banana, small	23.7	2.4	21.2	0.5	1.0	93
0.25	cup	Blackberries	4.6	1.9	2.7	0.1	0.3	19
0.25	cup	Blueberries	5.1	1.0	4.1	0.1	0.2	20
0.25	cup	Cantaloupe	3.3	0.3	3.0	0.1	0.4	14
0.25	cup	Cherries	4.8	0.7	4.2	0.3	0.4	21
0.25	cup	Cranberries, raw	3.0	1.0	2.0	0.0	0.1	12
0.25	cup	Currants, dried	26.7	2.4	24.2	0.1	1.5	102
0.25	cup	Dates, chopped	32.7	3.3	29.4	0.2	0.9	122
0.25	cup	Figs, dried	32.5	5.8	26.7	0.6	1.5	127
1.00	each	Figs, fresh	9.6	1.7	7.9	0.2	0.4	37
0.50	cup	Grapefruit Juice-Canned-Unsweet	9.2	1.4	7.9	0.1	0.7	37
0.25	cup	Grapes	7.1	0.4	6.7	0.2	0.3	28
0.25	cup	Honeydew Melon	3.9	0.3	3.6	0.0	0.2	15
0.50	cup	Juice, apple	14.5	0.1	14.4	0.1	0.1	58
0.50	cup	Juice, cranberry	18.2	0.1	18.1	0.1	0.0	72
0.50	cup	Juice, grape	18.9	0.1	18.8	0.1	0.7	77
0.50	cup	Juice, grapefruit	11.1	0.1	10.9	0.1	0.6	47
1.00	tbs	Juice, lemon	1.3	0.1	1.3	0.0	0.1	4

0.50	cup	Juice, orange	13.4	0.2	13.2	0.1	0.8	56
0.50	cup	Juice, tomato	5.1	0.5	4.7	0.1	0.9	21
1.00	each	Kiwifruit	11.3	2.6	8.7	0.3	0.8	46
0.25	cup	Mango	7.0	0.7	6.3	0.1	0.2	27
1.00	each	Nectarine	16.0	2.2	13.8	0.6	1.3	67
1.00	each	Orange	16.3	3.4	12.9	0.1	1.4	64
0.25	cup	Papaya	3.4	0.6	2.8	0.0	0.2	14
1.00	each	Peach, medium	10.9	2.0	8.9	0.1	0.7	42
1.00	each	Pear, medium	25.1	4.0	21.1	0.7	0.6	98
0.25	cup	Pineapple	4.8	0.5	4.3	0.2	0.2	19
1.00	each	Plums	8.6	1.0	7.6	0.4	0.5	36
0.25	cup	Prunes	26.7	3.0	23.6	0.2	1.1	102
0.25	cup	Raspberries	3.6	2.1	1.5	0.2	0.3	15
0.25	cup	Seedless Raisins	32.6	1.7	31.0	0.2	1.3	124
0.25	cup	Strawberries	2.7	0.9	1.8	0.1	0.2	11
1.00	each	Tangerine	7.8	1.6	6.2	0.1	0.4	31
0.25	cup	Watermelon	2.8	0.2	2.6	0.2	0.2	12

Food Item

			Total Carbs (g)	Fiber (g)	Net Carbs (g)	Fat (g)	Pro- tein	Calo- ries

Vegetables

			Total Carbs (g)	Fiber (g)	Net Carbs (g)	Fat (g)	Pro- tein	Calo- ries
1.00	each	Artichoke	13.4	6.5	6.9	0.2	4.2	60
1.00	each	Artichoke hearts, marinated	1.0	0.0	1.0	2.5	0.0	25
6.00	each	Asparagus spears	3.8	1.4	2.4	0.3	2.3	22
0.50	cup	Beans, green	4.9	2.0	2.9	0.2	1.2	22
1.00	cup	Bok Choy	1.5	0.7	0.8	0.1	1.1	9
0.50	cup	Broccoflower	3.1	1.6	1.5	0.2	1.5	16
0.50	cup	Broccoli	3.9	2.3	1.7	0.3	2.3	22
0.50	cup	Broccoli rabe	2.0	0.0	2.0	0.0	1.3	10
6.00	each	Brussels sprouts	10.9	3.3	7.6	0.6	3.2	49
0.50	cup	Cabbage, green	1.9	0.8	1.1	0.1	0.4	8
0.50	cup	Cabbage, red	1.9	0.8	1.1	0.1	0.5	9
0.50	cup	Cabbage, sauerkraut	5.1	3.0	2.1	0.2	1.1	22
0.50	cup	Cabbage, savoy	2.1	1.1	1.1	0.0	0.7	9
1.00	each	Carrots, medium	7.3	2.2	5.1	0.1	0.7	31
6.00	each	Cauliflower florets	4.4	2.9	1.5	0.5	2.0	25
1.00	each	Celery stalk (medium)	1.5	0.7	0.8	0.1	0.3	6
1.00	tbs	Celery, chopped	0.3	0.1	0.1	0.0	0.1	1
1.00	each	Chili Pepper	0.0	0.0	0.0	0.0	0.0	20
1.00	tbs	Chilies, green, chopped	0.5	0.5	0.0	0.0	0.0	3
4.00	oz-wt	Collards	7.3	4.1	3.2	0.4	3.1	37

1.00	each	Cucumber, English	4.0	1.1	2.8	0.3	0.9	19
0.50	each	Cucumber, small	2.5	0.7	1.8	0.2	0.6	12
0.50	cup	Daikon	1.8	0.7	1.1	0.0	0.3	8
0.50	cup	Eggplant	3.3	1.2	2.0	0.1	0.4	14
0.50	cup	Eggplant, Italian	3.3	1.2	2.0	0.1	0.4	14
0.50	cup	Endive	1.8	1.4	0.4	0.0	0.4	8
0.50	cup	Escarole	0.8	0.8	0.1	0.1	0.3	4
0.50	cup	Fennel	3.2	1.3	1.8	0.1	0.5	13
1.00	cup	Greens, mixed	1.6	1.2	0.4	0.1	0.9	9
0.50	cup	Jicama	5.7	3.2	2.5	0.1	0.5	25
0.50	cup	Kale	3.7	1.3	2.4	0.3	1.2	18
1.00	each	Leeks	12.6	1.6	11.0	0.3	1.3	54
1.00	cup	Lettuce, butterhead	1.3	0.6	0.7	0.1	0.7	7
1.00	cup	Lettuce, romaine	1.3	1.0	0.4	0.1	0.9	8
0.50	cup	Mushroom, portobello	1.4	0.4	1.0	0.1	1.0	9
2.00	tbs	Mushrooms, dried	8.9	2.9	6.0	0.7	5.6	64
0.50	cup	Mushrooms, fresh	1.4	0.4	1.0	0.1	1.0	9
4.00	oz-wt	Okra	7.5	2.5	5.0	0.3	1.9	34
1.00	each	Onions	9.5	2.0	7.5	0.2	1.3	42
0.25	cup	Onions, green	1.8	0.7	1.2	0.0	0.5	8
0.50	cup	Peas, edible podded	5.6	2.2	3.4	0.2	2.6	34
0.50	cup	Peas, green	9.9	3.4	6.5	0.3	3.8	55
0.50	cup	Pepper, green	4.8	1.3	3.4	0.1	0.7	20
0.50	cup	Pepper, red	4.8	1.5	3.3	0.1	0.7	20
1.00	each	Peppers, jalapeno	0.8	0.4	0.4	0.1	0.2	4
0.50	each	Peppers, roasted	2.4	0.4	2.0	0.1	0.3	10

			Total Carbs (g)	Fiber (g)	Net Carbs (g)	Fat (g)	Pro-tein	Calo-ries
0.50	cup	Potato, white	15.4	1.5	13.9	0.1	1.4	66
0.50	cup	Pumpkin	9.9	3.6	6.3	0.3	1.3	42
0.50	cup	Radicchio	0.9	0.2	0.7	0.1	0.3	5
6.00	each	Radishes	1.0	0.4	0.5	0.1	0.2	5
0.50	cup	Rhubarb	2.8	1.1	1.7	0.1	0.5	13
0.25	cup	Shallots	6.7	0.3	6.4	0.0	1.0	29
1.00	cup	Spinach, raw	1.1	0.8	0.2	0.1	0.9	7
0.50	cup	Squash, acorn	14.9	4.5	10.4	0.1	1.1	57

Food Item

			Total Carbs (g)	Fiber (g)	Net Carbs (g)	Fat (g)	Pro-tein	Calo-ries
0.50	cup	Squash, butternut	10.8	2.9	7.9	0.1	0.9	41
0.50	cup	Squash, spaghetti	5.0	1.1	3.9	0.2	0.5	21
0.50	cup	Squash, summer	2.5	1.1	1.4	0.1	0.7	11
1.00	each	Squash, zucchini	5.7	2.4	3.3	0.3	2.3	27
0.5	each	Sweet potato (medium)	13.8	1.7	12.1	1.0	0.1	62
0.50	cup	Swiss chard	0.7	0.3	0.4	0.0	0.3	3
1.00	each	Tomatillos	2.0	0.6	1.3	0.3	0.3	11
1.00	each	Tomato, plum	4.2	1.0	3.2	0.3	0.8	19
1.00	each	Tomato, small	4.2	1.0	3.2	0.3	0.8	19
0.50	cup	Tomatoes, canned	5.2	1.2	4.0	0.2	1.1	23
6.00	each	Tomatoes, cherry	4.7	1.1	3.6	0.3	0.9	21
0.50	cup	Tomatoes, chopped	3.5	0.8	2.6	0.2	0.6	16

			Total Carbs (g)	Fiber (g)	Net Carbs (g)	Fat (g)	Pro-tein	Calo-ries
0.25	cup	Tomatoes,	6.4	1.6	4.8	3.9	1.4	59
0.50	cup	Turnips	3.8	1.6	2.3	0.1	0.6	16
0.50	cup	Water chestnuts	8.7	1.8	7.0	0.0	0.6	35
0.50	cup	Watercress	0.2	0.2	0.0	0.0	0.4	2

Food Item

			Total Carbs (g)	Fiber (g)	Net Carbs (g)	Fat (g)	Pro-tein	Calo-ries
Alcohol								
12.00	fl oz	Beer	13.2	0.7	12.5	0.0	1.1	146
1.00	fl oz	Bourbon-80 Proof	0.0	0.0	0.0	0.0	0.0	64
1.00	oz-wt	Brandy-86 Proof	0.0	0.0	0.0	0.0	0.0	71
1.00	oz-wt	Brandy-86 Proof	0.0	0.0	0.0	0.0	0.0	71
1.00	oz-wt	Gin-80 Proof	0.0	0.0	0.0	0.0	0.0	65
4.00	fl oz	Medium White Wine	0.9	0.0	0.9	0.0	0.1	80
4.00	fl oz	Red Wine	2.0	0.0	2.0	0.0	0.2	85
1.00	oz-wt	Rum-80 Proof	0.0	0.0	0.0	0.0	0.0	65
1.00	oz-wt	Tequila-80 Proof	0.0	0.0	0.0	0.0	0.0	65
1.00	oz-wt	Triple Sec Liqueur-1 Shot	12.5	0.0	12.5	0.1	0.0	100
1.00	oz-wt	Vodka-80 Proof	0.0	0.0	0.0	0.0	0.0	65
1.00	oz-wt	Whiskey-80 Proof	0.0	0.0	0.0	0.0	0.0	65